# The NURSE'S GUIDE to
# SUCCESSFUL
# MANAGEMENT
## A Desk Reference

*Visit our website at* **www.mosby.com**

# The NURSE'S GUIDE to SUCCESSFUL MANAGEMENT

## A Desk Reference

**JO MCGUFFIN, PhD, RN, NMCC**
Director, Medical and Surgical Services
Eastern New Mexico Medical Center
Roswell, New Mexico

*with* **60** *illustrations*

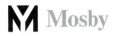 Mosby

St. Louis  Baltimore  Boston  Carlsbad
Chicago  Minneapolis  New York  Philadelphia  Portland
London  Milan  Sydney  Tokyo  Toronto

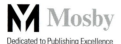 **Mosby**

Dedicated to Publishing Excellence

Publisher: Sally Schrefer
Editor: Yvonne Alexopoulos
Managing Editor: Lisa Potts
Developmental Editor: Aimee E. Loewe
Project Manager: Patricia Tannian
Senior Production Editor: Melissa Mraz Lastarria
Design Manager: Gail Morey Hudson
Manufacturing Buyer: Debbie Larocca
Cover Design: Teresa Breckwoldt

Composition by Carlisle Communications, Ltd.
Printing/binding by R.R. Donnelley & Sons Company

Mosby, Inc.
11830 Westline Industrial Drive
St. Louis, Missouri 63146

**International Standard Book Number 0-323-00388-5**

99  00  01  02  03  /  9  8  7  6  5  4  3  2  1

# Contributors

**C. DANIEL GORMAN**
Corporate Human Resource Specialist

**VIVIEN JUTSUM, RN, MSN, CS**
Education Specialist
Heartland Health System
St. Joseph, Missouri

**SANDRA PIERSON**
Healthcare Human Resource Specialist

# Reviewers

**JANE CAMPBELL, RN, MSN, CNA**
Associate Professor
Northern Michigan University
Marquette, Michigan
Home Health Care Private Duty Consultant
Marquette County Health Department
Negaunee, Michigan

**LARRY DALE TAZAN PURNELL, MSN, PhD, RN**
Associate Professor
College of Health and Nursing Sciences
University of Delaware
Newark, Delaware
Professor, Administration
University of Panama
Republic of Panama

**BARBARA V. CLYDE, MS, RN**
Vice President Nursing
Comanche County Memorial Hospital
Lawton, Oklahoma

**BILLIE R. ROZELL, DSN, RN**
Associate Professor
College of Nursing
The University of Alabama in Huntsville
Huntsville, Alabama

**SUSAN M. WELLS, RN, MS**
Healthcare Consultant
Lexington Kentucky
Research Associate
College of Nursing
University of Kentucky
Lexington, Kentucky
Doctoral Student
Health and Organizational Communications
University of Kentucky
Lexington, Kentucky

# Preface

Managers in healthcare today are facing new complexities in scope and scale. They encounter new relationships and responsibilities and frequently work within multi-provider arrangements. As a result, managers cannot ignore the interests of physicians, contract employers, consumers, and insurers. In addition, the boundaries within which healthcare is organized, financed, evaluated, and modified are becoming increasingly blurred and difficult to decipher. Amidst this changing environment, administrators must continue to develop themselves, as well as orient and precept other healthcare managers who possess varying levels of experience and skills.

*The Nurse's Guide to Successful Management: A Desk Reference* presents the "nuts and bolts" of practical management concepts and subsequent sample tools essential for any healthcare setting. This book facilitates sound managerial competencies and problem-solving skills and can be used as an excellent tool for teaching instruction and decision support. The generic management tools provided assist managers in organization, fiscal and administrative management, and data collection and analysis. These tools can be easily modified for specific environments and dimensions of performance to best fit your needs.

Essential leadership and management concepts for multi-level management and executive positions have been consolidated throughout this book. The topics covered include frequently requested information and the perceived needs for nurse leaders related to the changing healthcare environment. Each chapter completely and concisely addresses a specific topic vital to the nurse management role:

- Chapter 1, *Leadership,* explores leadership values and attributes that ensure success and promote increased intellectual, emotional, and professional maturity.
- Chapter 2, *Human Resource Principles,* addresses the essentials of the hiring process, which helps you effectively and efficiently recruit the right person. In addition, this chapter serves as a reference guide to assist you through essential documentation and regulatory guidelines of personnel management.
- Chapter 3, *Management Principles,* details problem-solving models and methods for analyzing alternatives with the help of analytical tools used for organizing, planning, and decision making.
- Chapter 4, *Quality and Productivity,* contains multiple sample tools used operationally in various healthcare settings to help you efficiently manage without "reinventing the wheel."
- Chapter 5, *Networking Skills,* introduces essential skills and tips necessary for effective networking.
- Chapter 6, *Marketing Skills,* walks you through the strategic planning process and marketing orientation so that you understand each step involved in the development of both strategic and marketing plans.
- Chapter 7, *Politics for the Healthcare Manager,* tackles the pitfalls and challenges of "playing politics" in the healthcare field with practical guidelines.
- Chapter 8, *Managed Care,* explores this growing segment in today's healthcare arena and provides you with specific "must know" information.
- Chapter 9, *Competency-Based Education,* thoroughly explains competency-based educations so that you can conceptualize competency versus competence and be able to develop and implement a competency-based education program within any organization.
- Appendices contain valuable tools, reporting formats, competency standards, and performance improvement examples that you can use on the job and photocopy for future use.

In addition, special features have been included and high-lighted throughout the text. *Action Tips* boxes concisely sum up key management skills and provide practical, step-by-step ideas for application. *Management Spotlight* boxes focus on specific tips and thoughts for nurse managers. Chapter quotes from well-known and respected sources introduce each chapter.

My contributors and I worked to *operationalize* the essentials of various concepts by providing appropriate tools you can readily use to help develop your management skills and function more effectively in your position. The material and references were carefully selected to provide the most comprehensive coverage of these topics. As you will find, many of the references listed are outside the nursing discipline and, in some cases, outside the healthcare industry. These references combine the "classics" and most current management resources available.

I believe you will find this book a valuable reference for managers in varying levels of practice and experience.

**Jo McGuffin**

# Acknowledgments

Few works are written as solos. Behind the words I have pulled together lies the works and deeds of a full chorus of voices. In addition to the voices I have listened to in a lifetime of reading, are the voices of special people who have cared enough to push me, challenge me, counsel me, and love me.

My mother, *Emilie,* is a woman who always had time to listen, inspire, and love me. My father, *Bill,* taught me to put the Lord Jesus Christ first in my life and let Him faithfully direct my footsteps.

My beloved husband, *Stephen,* whom I adore, has given me unselfish support, inspiration, unconditional love, and encouragement to exceed my own expectations. Thank you for being my partner and best friend.

My wonderful children serve the Lord with gladness and joy. They are every mom's dream of what kids can be with their gentle spirits and loving kindness that allows everyone to see the Father's heart in them.

My in-laws, *Barbara* and *Melvin,* accept me unconditionally as their own. I am so blessed to have yet another place to call home.

The publishing staff at Mosby whose propulsion brought this idea into reality. My appreciation goes to the editorial staff and reviewers who spent endless hours assisting me with the final product.

To these and many friends and colleagues whose names do not appear here but are carved on my heart, I give you my grateful thanks.

And last, but certainly not least, I give all the glory, honor, and praise to you Lord Jesus. Amazing grace! Thank you for teaching me, leading me, and loving me.

# Contents

# Part One
# Leadership
# Responsibilities

# Chapter 1

# Leadership

*Life afforts no greater responsibility, no greater privilege, than raising of the next generation.*

*Deuteronomy 11:19-21 NIV*

## LEADERS VERSUS MANAGERS

Managers are a dime a dozen, but leaders are still premium assets to healthcare organizations. Old habits and attitudes must be consigned to the past, making way for emergent leaders plugged into inspiring visions and future-oriented attitudes. Managers coordinate staffing needs, manage inventories and supplies, collect data, and crunch numbers. True leaders act as role models, set transcendent goals, develop people, and expect excellence.

Pronouncements of *dedicated to service* and *committed to excellence* are not enough and such claims are often counterproductive in organization where action plans are conspicuous by their absence. Such rhetoric without demonstrable follow through and strategic thrust, creates disillusionment in customers, as well as employees.

Swansburg (1990) differentiates leadership as a desirable feature of the directing function of nursing management. Managers are delegated authority and are expected to perform in the basic functions of management: planning, organizing, directing, and controlling.

Successful managers problem solve, analyze results, and are usually appointed for both technical and management competencies. Managers who are leaders choose specific goals and focus on developing people; subsequently they then develop followers. Leaders seek advice and solutions to problems from networking, benchmarking, and empowering constituents to formulate solutions. People are challenged to stretch their potentials.

Leaders are distinguished beyond the general run of managers in the following six respects (Swansburg, 1990):

- Leaders think longer-term; beyond the horizon.
- Leaders look beyond the unit or department and look to its relationship with the organizational strategic priorities, cues from the external environment and global trends.
- Leaders influence constituents and colleagues beyond their scope of responsibility; go beyond bureaucratic boundaries; dissolve fragmentation.
- Leaders emphasize the intangibles of vision, values, and motivation. They understand the underlying dynamics of a culture and are able to still influence, regardless of barriers and sometimes adverse dynamics.
- Leaders think in terms of continuous performance improvement; challenging systems, processes, and structures.
- Leaders develop political skill and stamina to cope with conflicting requirements of multiple stakeholders.

Swansburg (1990) further asserts that effective nurse executives combine leadership and management. He describes five major requirements for every executive that imply that the executive position should require attributes of a leader.

- Adaptable to a complex social environment of many services.
- Ability to influence and develop subordinates.
- Emotional, intellectual, and professional maturity as preparatory for leadership.
- Analytic decision making and ability to translate into effective action.
- Capacity to see beyond the symptoms, surface indications, and perceptions, and acquires perspective.

## LEADERSHIP BY EXPECTATION

Leadership by expectation is a relatively new style of management in terms of the longevity of the majority of leadership theories. This style of leadership requires fundamental changes in management attitudes. Leadership by expectation simply means to *become what we expect.* According to Batten (1989) there is a direct link between what we expect from ourselves and our team members, and what we and they actually achieve in terms of results that contribute directly to the company's profits.

Leadership by expectation anticipates the best from each person and gives them goals to reach only if they are prepared to stretch. It then holds individuals accountable for results and rewards performance that contributes to the corporate goals. Individuals are not viewed in organizational boxes, nor are they directed and pushed into meeting goals as with traditional styles. Leaders set the example by their own attitudes and role-modeling.

Leadership by expectation goes beyond *Management by Objectives* (MBO), in that it is mutually understood that to get the best results a manager must do more than merely establish goals and objectives. People must be involved and subsequently committed to the goals. Leaders must be willing to invest the time to identify and develop a real understanding of the drives and ambitions of each team member and encourage that potential in each person. According to Batten (1989), this then results in the synergistic effect needed to increase productivity of the team. Batten further asserts that control does not come from the outside; it is the self-control that comes from enlightened, involved, and committed people working together as a team. He makes an analogy of ordinary light and laser light. The only difference is the focus and intensity.

Leadership by expectation requires that the leader develop a certain toughness that is the hallmark of Batten's tough-minded leadership. Expectations are much stronger than directives and subsequently yield much greater results. However, for many managers and executives, it is easier to give directives or not get involved much at all. The latter characteristic is observed in managers and executives who have encouraged an environment or culture of complacency or status quo. It takes enormous energy to lead by expectation. It requires courage to take risks, to change attitudes, to cause unsettling within the status quo. An example of leadership by expectation is observed in a corporation called IBM. The company enjoys success from building on strengths, rather than focusing on employee weaknesses. The most important belief is the respect for the individual that is the foundation of the philosophy, the spirit, and the drive of the organization.

To build on strengths, a manager must first identify both the existing and potential strengths of each individual. When the departmental goals and performance standards are developed, challenge employees to meet stretching goals based on their identified strengths. Reinforce these strengths, and expect excellence. Hold each person accountable for results and reward them accordingly. Continuous feedback (and compensation when feasible) based on results will foster a climate of motivation to meet those goals and improve performance.

Since performance is based on people, performance improves only when people improve. Well-written standards of performance must be specific: required results defined and how measured. Goals should be progressively targeted at stretching the horizon and raising the bar toward excellence. The goals then provide validity for positive reinforcement.

True leaders are confident that authority does not come from the position, but from the example set daily and quality of actions. The real leader serves others by being the catalyst to develop people to grow, mature, and thrive. The true leader expects excellence from self and others.

## Strong Leadership Enhances Productivity

Much of the management literature centers around the management process: plan, execute, coordinate, and control.

## Management Spotlight

*POINTS TO PONDER FOR PRESIDENTS*
*(AND OTHER MANAGERS)*

Even the most powerful lose effectiveness as soon as one of these rules are violated:

1. One first must ask, "What needs to be done?"; then begin to prioritize and implement changes.
2. Concentrate, don't splinter yourself.
3. Don't ever bet on a sure thing.
4. A president has no friends in administration.
5. An effective leader does not micromanage.
6. Once elected, stop campaigning. (Truman gave this advice to newly elected John F. Kennedy.)

From Drucker, P. (1995). *Managing in a time of change.* New York: Truman Tally Books/Dulton.

These may be the foundational elements; however, expective leadership goes beyond the process to develop the strengths, talents, and minds of people. Lance Secrtan (1997), in his book *Reclaiming Higher Ground,* emphasizes that true leaders create environments that inspire and motivate people. Creating this type of environment improves productivity. Japanese productivity methods identify core values to their management approach. Examples of the core values include spiritual values and fitness, which become integral parts of the organizational philosophy, policies, and practices.

A true leader cares about people enough to search out their strengths and best possibilities. Batten (1989) lists eight steps to foster a climate of heightened productivity.

1. Identify strengths that all team members show in work situations. Ask each member to list his or her own; tie strengths directly to job contributions.

2. Classify these strengths in three categories: decision making or evaluation, problem solving or analysis, and interpersonal relationship skills.

3. Develop these strengths through challenging assignments that stretch, combined with outside courses/continuing education.

4. Assign strengths where they will benefit the organization the most. Do not be boxed in by traditional roles. Identify which people can best meet which goal. Batten suggests that each manager keep a computerized log of each individual's list of strengths.

5. Set high expectations through mutually agreed on performance objectives. Then hold each person accountable for results. Blend personal goals with corporate goals to achieve a synergistic effect.

6. Measure strengths and monitor progress made toward goals. Recognize improvement, no matter how small or incremental.

7. Use feedback and self-control by each person to keep performance levels high. Compensate, if feasible, for results produced. In healthcare settings, financial compensation is not always possible; therefore creative ways must be used to positively reward and acknowledge people for positive results.

8. Give complete primacy to strong and focused minds.

A very successful company in America, the Marriot Corporation, utilizes Batten's tough-minded leadership principles. They also share core values, and the development of people is viewed as a priority. The essence of their beliefs is depicted in the following published guideposts for the corporation (Batten, 1989):

1. Keep physically fit, mentally and spiritually strong.

2. Guard your habits; bad ones will destroy you.

3. Pray about every difficult problem.

4. Study and follow professional management principles. Apply them logically to your organization.

5. People are number one—their growth, loyalty, interest, team spirit. Develop managers in every area. This is your prime responsibility.

6. Decisions: Men and women grow while making decisions and assuming responsibility for them.
   A. Make crystal clear what decision each manager is responsible for and what decisions you reserve for yourself.
   B. Have all the facts and counsel necessary—then decide and stick to it.
7. Criticism: Do not criticize people, but make a fair appraisal of their qualifications with their supervisor only (or someone assigned to do this).
8. See the best in people and try to develop those qualities.
9. Inefficiency: If it cannot be overcome and an employee is obviously incapable of the job, find a job that he or she can do or terminate now. Do not wait.
10. Manage your time.
    A. Keep conversations short and to the point.
    B. Make every minute on the job count.
11. Delegate and hold accountable for results.
12. Details:
    A. Let your staff take care of themselves.
    B. Save your energy for planning, proposals, analysis of data, contributing in meetings, special projects.
13. Ideas and Competition:
    A. Ideas keep the business alive.
    B. Know what your competitors are doing and planning.
    C. Encourage all managers to think about better ways and give suggestions on anything that will improve business.
    D. Spend time and money on research and development.
14. Do not try to do an employee's job for him or her; counsel and suggest.
15. Think objectively and keep a sense of humor. Make the business fun for you and others.

## Tough-Minded Leadership

Leadership is truly needed in management today. A company's profit and future are only as strong as the corporate culture. To become a culture of excellence can only be envisioned and created by leaders of excellence. Batten's (1989) *tough-minded leadership* principles are superior guidelines for transforming from the traditional view of leadership to the expectation view of leadership (Box 1-1).

True leaders practice their personal values. Last, but not least, Batten (1989) reflects values that should be believed and practiced daily as a *tough-minded leader:*

1. Openness and emotional vulnerability. The absence of defensiveness is an indication of strength and management maturity.
2. Warmth. Leaders reach out to people.
3. Consistency. Leaders meet commitments, keep their word, and are reliable.
4. Unity. Leaders demonstrate oneness of purpose, effort, and direction.
5. Caring. Leaders get personal satisfaction when others grow and benefit.
6. Positive listening. Leaders keep a positive and open mind. They hear.
7. Unsatisfaction. Leaders want continuous improvement; they challenge systems, processes, and procedures. They constantly stretch for the best.
8. Flexibility. Leaders do not favor rigidity.
9. Giving. Leaders believe that giving yields real pleasure.
10. Involvement. Leaders seek involvement from their constituents.
11. Tolerance of mistakes. Leaders have the courage to let people make mistakes.
12. Values. Leaders perceive values as precision instruments to inspire, motivate, and stretch.
13. Psychological wages. Leaders provide for positive feedback.
14. Simplicity. Leaders view that settling for a complex solution is settling for second best.
15. Time. Leaders guard their time preciously and allot it to key areas with the greatest impact.

## BOX 1-1

# MAKING THE TOUGH-MINDED TRANSITION

| From | To |
| --- | --- |
| Directiveness | Expectiveness |
| Compromising expectations | Clear, stretching expectations |
| Defensiveness | Open, warm, thoughtful candor |
| Activity documents and reports | Performance progress reports |
| Hunch and guess | Disciplined, researched decisions |
| Inconsistency and emotionalism | Consistency and focus |
| Conformity and rebellion | Individuality and competing with self |
| Competing with others | Competing with self |
| Complexity | Simplicity |
| Dialogue (two or more engaged in monologues) | Communication (shared understanding) |
| Procrastination | Confrontation |
| Euphemism | Specificity |
| Crises and fire fighting | Identify early warning systems |
| Office politics and defensiveness | Team synergy and openness |
| Blurred, expedient morality | Tough, stretching moral practices |
| Reaction to symptoms | Proaction dealing with cause |
| Disparate actions | Unifying team actions |
| Compensation based on actions and personal characteristics | Compensation based on positive performance |
| Fragmentation and diffusion of effort | Purpose and direction |
| Getting | Giving |
| Focusing on weaknesses | Building on strengths |
| Commitment to self only | Commitment to goals and objectives that transcend self |
| Guarded behavior | Caring and giving |
| Negative listening | Positive listening |
| Dissatisfaction (past-oriented) | Unsatisfaction (future-oriented) |
| Gamesmanship | Accountability for results |
| Expecting the worst | Expecting the best |

From Batten, J. (1989). *Tough-minded leadership.* New York: American Management Association.

16. The winning formula: Integrity + quality + service.
17. An open mind. An open mind can grow.
18. Development of people. Leaders believe and live this concept. The development of people pays great dividends to both the organization and the individual.
19. Self-discipline. Leaders practice in all dimensions of life.
20. Physical fitness. Leaders recognize that this is an obligation to a business. Physical fitness is an important requisite of mental health and acuity.
21. Enjoyment of life. Leaders enjoy life—are pleasant, cheerful. They enjoy work.
22. Broad perspective. Leaders read widely and have personal development programs and goals.
23. Faith in self and others. Leaders believe that all have worth and contributions.
24. Vision. Vision provides the basis of energy, framework, and stretch for moving the organization forward.
25. Positive thinking. Leaders believe negativism is never justified.
26. Desire to learn. Leaders cultivate desires for new dimensions of knowledge.
27. Integrity. Leaders know that there is no substitute; they live integrity.
28. Results, not activity. Excellent leaders measure performance in terms of results and their contributions to the organization.
29. Candor. Leaders practice truth rigorously; they are truthful, yet gracious, with colleagues.
30. Management by example. Leaders believe that actions of responsible leaders are contagious.
31. A clear philosophy, purpose, and direction. Leaders ensure that the philosophy and objectives are researched, developed, and clearly communicated.
32. Accountability. Leaders believe people are more efficient and positive when clear parameters are understood.
33. Purpose and direction. Leaders are visionaries.
34. Expectation of excellence. Leaders raise the standards and expect positive results.

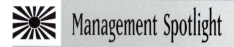

## Management Spotlight

### BE A GOOD SPORT

Good Sports:

- Promote harmony
- Play fair . . . show respect for others instead of putting someone down
- Demonstrate humility . . . big enough to admit mistakes and say "I'm sorry"
- Demonstrate grace . . . Forgiving teammates when foul-ups occur, and sharing the spotlight when one does well.

Moments of truth occur daily when one doesn't get own way; when one is under pressure.

From Pritchett, P. (1997). *The team member handbook for teamwork.* Dallas: Pritchett & Associates.

Joe Batten is a leadership *giant* in and has made unique contributions to organizational and individual development. The following *commandments* epitomize Batten's (1989) *tough-minded* leadership principles:

### The Ten Commandments of Expective Leadership

1. I will *tell* no one. But I will *expect* much.
2. The truth is the only thing that sets you free.
3. I will diligently expect to *be* what I expect of others.
4. I will unleash, unshackle, and be proud of my enthusiasm.
5. I will search for some positive strengths in every person. I will expect each person's best.
6. I will share life, love, and laughter with my team.
7. I know that expectations are the key to all happenings.
8. I know that the best control is a clearly and mutually understood expectation.
9. I will sculpt a vision and plan boldly.
10. I will *live* my plan. I will *lead* my team.

## LEADERSHIP IN A VALUE-DRIVEN ORGANIZATION

Healthcare organizations are now value driven: providing quality care cost effectively. Leaders must now be transformational rather than the traditional transactional. Transactional leadership is usually episodic and limited to an exchange transaction (or resource valued by the follower) such as a paycheck. Transformational leadership is complex and occurs when both the leaders and followers raise one another to higher levels of motivation and ethical aspiration. The following descriptions depict ways to lead in a value driven organization (Starkweather & Shropshire, 1994):

**Communicating a Vision.** The effective manager must inspire others by articulating a clear vision for the organization or individual department. This must be done in such a way that staff become excited by the vision and begin to develop a "can do" attitude.

**Commitment to the Development of Others.** The effective manager creates an environment in which employees can become successful. Managing others often equates to managing the development of others. In this new era, an effective leader becomes a coach, a teacher, and a mentor for others. An essential focus will be to optimize the strengths of others while strengthening the weaknesses of the leader.

**Establishing Values.** It is the leader's role to declare what the organization/department stands for, establish the standard of practice for all to achieve, and communicate these standards clearly. Managing the transformation of an organization's culture is the process of establishing values. With any standard, it is important for the self-esteem and respect of others to know that behavior and performance are being evaluated in the context of a value system. "Principled leadership" is reinforcing the established system of values by personal example.

**Learning.** Drucker (1995) proposes that managers have to learn to ask critical questions of every process, every product, every policy. In addition, transformational leaders draw on three systematic practices:

1. Continuing improvement of everything the organization does.
2. Every organization will have to learn to expand its knowledge to develop next generation applications from its own successes.
3. Every organization must learn to innovate, redesign, transform.

Senge (1990) illustrates a vision of the future that he described as the "learning organization." He describes systems thinking, personal mastery, mental models, building a shared vision and team learning as essential disciplines in the learning organization. Senge goes on to describe leaders as *designers, teachers,* and *stewards.* Healthcare environments, both external and internal, are constantly changing; therefore opportunities must be provided for managers at all levels to gain new knowledge.

**Establishing Priorities and Directions.**  Leadership establishes the strategic direction and subsequently focuses the organization's initiatives on addressing its priorities.

**Solving Problems.**  The effective leader can differentiate core problems from symptoms of underlying problems. In addition, the effective manager analyzes the effectiveness of all the potential solutions and the potential impact of implementation of those solutions on all departments. Decisions from an effective leader are then based on the best initiative that is congruent with the organizational strategic objectives. As managers and subordinates learn to utilize tools to assist them in problem-solving methodologies, the easier it is for employees to sense empowerment to solve problems at the point of service.

**Balancing Interests.** The effective manager works to balance the interests of all the organizational stakeholders, usually to the benefit of the strategic priorities. Often skills in negotiation, facilitation, and conflict resolution are utilized.

**Working for the Public Benefit.**  In most organizations, the community and patient benefits are priority objectives; however, other objectives must be somewhat balanced (value-driven).

Leadership

**Revising Traditional Leadership and Management Approaches.**
Leaders and managers must shift from exclusive strategic
planning to sharing mission/vision strategies and planning.
Leaders must shift from minimizing risks to mastering change.
Leaders must shift from maximizing profits to serving the
customers (Rowland, 1994).

Boxes 1-2 and 1-3 reflect characteristics of the manager
versus nurse executive as viewed by different authors and
frames of reference. It is interesting to note that many leadership attributes are those needed for all level positions.

---

**BOX 1-2**

## CHARACTERISTICS OF THE
## SUCCESSFUL MANAGER

**Intellectual Functioning**
- *Creativity.* Ability to generate, recognize, and/or accept imag-
  inative solutions and innovations.
- *Risk Taking.* Ability to weigh alternatives and make decisions
  in which a calculated risk is taken to achieve maximum benefits.
- *Problem Analysis.* Ability to identify and weigh alternatives to
  specified problems.
- *Judgment.* Ability to make a considered decision.
- *Decisiveness.* Ability to make a decision in a timely fashion.
- *Financial Analysis.* Ability to understand the financial impact
  of various occurrences and circumstances.
- *Common Sense.* Ability to make the right decision in
  untimely situations.

**Emotional Functioning**
- *Stress Tolerance.* Stability of performance under pressure and
  opposition.
- *Initiative.* Actively influences events rather than passively accepting; self-starting; takes action beyond what is necessarily called
  for; originates actions rather than just responding to events.
- *Tenacity.* Tendency to stay with a problem or line of thought
  until the matter is resolved; perseverance.
- *Resilience.* Ability to bounce back after difficult and trying
  circumstances.

**BOX 1-2—cont'd**

**Communication**
- *Adaptability.* Ability to maintain effectiveness in different situations and handle changing responsibilities.
- *Listening Skills.* Ability to extract important information in oral communications.
- *Oral and Written Communication Skills.* Effectiveness of expression clearly and correctly.

**Insight into Self and Others**
- *Development of Subordinates and Self.* Ability to recognize own strengths and weaknesses and those of subordinates; ability to utilize strengths of all members of team and take creative action to effect needed behavior change.
- *Openness.* Willingness to accept feedback from others in a nondefensive manner.

**Management of Self and Others**
- *Flexibility.* Ability to modify behavioral style and management approach to reach a goal.
- *Organizational Sensitivity.* Skill in perceiving the impact and implications of decisions on other components of the organization.
- *Planning and Organization.* Ability to establish an appropriate course of action for self and/or others to accomplish a specific goal efficiently; ability to make proper assignments of personnel and appropriate use of resources.
- *Management Control.* Skill in establishing procedures to monitor (or regulate) processes, tasks, or activities of subordinates; ability to evaluate the results of delegated assignments and projects.
- *Use of Delegation.* Ability to work effectively with care managers and subordinate staff and understand at what level a decision can be made.
- *Political Sensitivity.* Awareness of changing societal and government pressures from outside the organization.

Modified from Spitzer-Lehmann, R. (1989). 'Middle Management' Consolidation, *Nursing Management,* Vol. 20:8. In H. Rowland & B. Rowland (Eds.). *Nursing administration manual.* Rockville, MD: Aspen Publishing.

**BOX 1-3**

# LEADERSHIP ATTRIBUTES OF NURSE EXECUTIVES

According to the opinions from 2,500 healthcare leaders nationally surveyed, the top six transformational competencies and values required for leading the future healthcare organization are: mastering change, systems thinking, shared vision, continuous quality improvement, redefining healthcare, and serving the public/community (Wolford, et al, 1992). Effective leaders are also obtaining greater knowledge in healthcare policy, healthcare finance, healthcare research, and medical care systems. The effective leader has the following qualities:

- Influences the practice environment by stressing the importance of creating an environment in which the professional can participate collaboratively at both the organizational and professional levels.
- Serves as an emissary for nursing with the medical staff, the board, hospital administrators, and the public.
- Has uncompromised value systems, such as honesty, integrity, equity, trust, and compassion, accompanied by a drive for higher standards and a vision of excellence.
- Is a creative visionary and willing to take risks to master change.
- Demonstrates flexibility, adaptability, and marketability.
- Clearly articulates and disseminates information appropriately, maintaining excellent interpersonal skills.
- Challenges processes, asking critical questions in an attempt to stimulate others to think differently than the status quo.
- Directs subordinates to goal achievement; motivates staff to demonstrate quality outcomes.
- Teaches and trains staff; however, often serves as facilitator, mentor, and role model.
- Develops a sense of timing, then confidently proceeds with decision making and subsequent implementation of initiatives.
- Takes cues from the external environment and proactively implements value-driven changes.
- Constantly demonstrates professional growth by learning from others and listening to understand, not respond. Stays current and self-managed.

**BOX 1-3 — cont'd**

- Develops healthcare administration/business skills, including an understanding of fiscal and personnel management, systems thinking, strategic planning and marketing, and healthcare politics.
- Expands professional interests outside of work environment to influence the community, professional organizations, and governmental policy.
- Looks for improvement opportunities; takes the initiative to champion new project developments.

Modified from Rowland, H. & Rowland, B. (1995). *Nursing administration manual.* Rockville, MD: Aspen Publishers.

## COMPETENCIES FOR THE SENIOR EXECUTIVE IN INTEGRATED DELIVERY SYSTEMS

As a result of healthcare changes, senior healthcare managers in integrated delivery systems (IDS), need different skills and knowledge (competencies) than managers within an independent healthcare organization. These managers work differently than their predecessors in independent organizations and, according to Longest (1998), clusters of knowledge and skills make up the appropriate competencies for this level of manager.

The senior managers in IDS environments are involved in managing a spectrum of services spanning the life cycles of the people in the populations served. Another difference is the fact that senior managers in IDSs are accountable for the overall health status of the populations they serve. Senior managers in independent healthcare organizations are usually responsible only for outcomes achieved in the provision of their organizations specific services, but not the overall health status of the population.

Further differences are related to the complexity and financial arrangements of the networks. IDSs are formed to position themselves to assume fiscal accountability, more often under capitated arrangements. This forces the senior manager to engage heavily in complex analytical activities in response to imposed risks related to various financial arrangements. An example would be the evaluation of physician and patient care services practice patterns, efficiency, utilization, and risk management issues across a much broader scope of responsibility. Because IDSs are composed of multiple organizations under multiple collaborative arrangements, the mere management of the network becomes complex.

Longest (1998) further proposes six distinct competencies that are important for the success of senior managers in IDSs. The clusters of knowledge and skills that make up the competencies are: (1) conceptual, (2) technical managerial/clinical, (3) interpersonal/collaborative, (4) political, (5) commercial, and (6) governance. Many aspects of these clusters also interface with senior managers of independent health organizations; however, the importance and complexity in application are magnified greatly by increasing levels of integration.

### Conceptual Competence

Conceptual competence requires the individual to possess global vision for the organization and society at large. It involves the visualization of the complex interrelationships that exist among both people and resources. The ability to visualize all the complex interrelationships, and the ability to understand and interact with all the major stakeholders and individual cultures, is critical to the success of the corporate or senior level manager of the IDS.

### Technical Managerial/Clinical Competence

The domain of technical managerial/clinical competence requires strategic planning and business skills related to planning new services or redesigning services, designing programs, or arranging the financing of services. Increasingly popular preparation includes the MBA or health management graduate degree programs.

### Interpersonal/Collaborative Competence

The core elements of interpersonal/collaborative competence involve management development; motivating employees; articulating and communicating the system's philosophy, core values, vision, mission and objectives; negotiating contracts; and outcomes management. The measure of success is defined differently. Instead of an organization's revenue and market share as elements of success, the network senior manager would view objectives relating to enhancement of the health status of defined populations and integrating functions within the system.

### Political Competence

Political competence is defined, according to Longest (1998), as the dual capability to accurately assess the impact of public policies on the performance of their domains of responsibility and to influence public policymaking at both state and federal levels. He further asserts that senior managers in IDSs possess positional, reward, and expertise-based opportunities to influence public policymaking.

### Commercial Competence

Commercial competence reflects the ability of senior managers to establish and operate value-creating situations in which economic exchanges between buyers and sellers occur. Value in healthcare services requires that buyers and sellers of these services think about both the quality and the price of services. This skill is associated with both identifying and positioning an IDS in its markets and establishing strategies that enhance the IDS's ability to compete effectively in markets.

## Governance Competence

Healthcare organizations rely on senior managers to work in concert to establish a clear vision, to foster a culture that supports the realization of the vision, to lead the organization through various challenges, and to ensure the proper accountability to the organization's multiple stakeholders. The senior manager is usually part of the governing boards and needs to be able to develop and assist other executives and managers in governance responsibilities.

A basic control question for IDSs is whether governance should be centralized or decentralized. Longest (1998) lists three models currently used; none has emerged as a best practice model.

1. Corporate or System Board model: involves a completely centralized system-wide governing board.
2. Parent Holding Company model: decentralizes control and involves a corporate or system governing board and separate, subordinate boards at the level of component organizations in the system or network that share control with the corporate board.
3. Modified Holding Company model: a variation of parent holding company model, there is a system-wide governing board, but there are advisory boards for the component organizations instead of governing boards.

## SYSTEMS THINKING

According to organizational redesign consultant, Alain Gauthier (1996), the only way healthcare leaders can deal with the complexity and turbulence of rapid change is by using systems thinking. He further asserts systems thinking is a view of the world radically different from the traditional reactive-top-down management perspective.

The organizations that use systems thinking are learning organizations and leaders see the interrelationships with all the parts making up the whole. Leaders using systems thinking do not react to events with short-term solutions, they solve problems by analyzing the organization's underlying patterns and processes.

Organizations that operate with quick-fixes for crisis management fail to get at the underlying cause of the problem. Learning organization leaders are willing to take the long view and not trade off long-term performance improvement for short-term goals. Gauthier (1996) explored how leaders can shift their thinking and thus the performance of their own organizations. In addition, leaders in learning organizations, demonstrate inquiry: the willingness to test assumptions, ask difficult questions, and challenge beliefs.

Gauthier (1996) proposed new roles for healthcare leaders as they transform their organizations into learning organizations:

### Leaders' New Roles

- Midwife — The leader helps others give birth to their visions.
- Custodian — The leader serves as a steward to preserve the organization's vision.
- Gardener — The leader helps others grow and helps others voice views.
- Designer — The leader serves as the architect of new processes and structures.
- Learner/Listener/ Researcher — The leader is a life long learner, receptive and willing to change based on results of research.

## EFFECTIVE LEADERSHIP COMMUNICATION

Communication is simply shared meaning; shared understanding. For successful relationships and successful job performance, communication is critical. Batten (1989) describes nine elusive elements that are found in truly effective relationships and they play a vital role in effective communication. The nine elements include the following:

1. *Vulnerability*   Real leaders have the courage to become vulnerable. This takes self-confidence and integrity to really get involved with strengthening and growing in relationships.

2. *Openness*    The capacity to interact free of self-defeating defensiveness, increases steadily as we confront stretching objectives, difficulties, and possibilities.
3. *Positive Listening*    The desire to cultivate and develop listening skills to genuinely hear what a team member is saying, as well as feeling.
4. *Kinesics*    The ability to go beyond body language and not misread or prejudge based on a stereotype.
5. *High Expectations*    It is crucial to ensure that each person feels significant and that the manager is not acting preoccupied or ignoring another individual.
6. *Avoiding Judgments*    Do not search for and fixate on an individual's weaknesses. Instead, the manager should maximize the strengths.
7. *Reinforcement*    Positive reinforcement means to build on the strengths of individuals with new rewards, affirmations, and greater responsibilities.
8. *Caring*    Care enough to listen positively and challenge all policies, practices, and systems.
9. *Integrity*    Integrity is not only honest, but whole. Integrity is essential. Without integrity, there is no credibility and no communication.

### Becoming A Better Communicator

Communication is a skill that can always be improved. Communication skills can be developed by becoming a better listener, learning a few helpful responding styles, and avoiding common causes of communication breakdown (Chitty, 1993).

### *Listening*

Active listening and open posture are methods of communicating interest and attention. Nurses have difficulty listening because of a variety of reasons, namely preoccupation with tasks still yet to be done. Managers have common listening faults: interruption, finishing sentences for others, and lack of interest (Chitty, 1993).

*Responding Techniques*
*Empathy*   Consists of awareness, sensitivity, and identification with the feelings of others.
*Open-ended Questions*   Question that causes other person to answer fully, more than a simple yes or no.
*Giving Information*   Provide accurate information; take the opportunity to teach. However, do not give opinions; opinions are not usually helpful.
*Reflection*   Reflection implies respect. This is a method to encourage individual to problem solve and think through own actions.
*Silence*   Silence is usually considered uncomfortable. However, many times, to establish or preserve relationships, silence may be the only neutral option to keep emotions in check.

## Avoiding Common Causes of Communication Breakdown

*Failing to see the uniqueness of the individual.* This is usually due to preconceived ideas, prejudices, and stereotypes.
*Failure to recognize levels of meaning.* People often give verbal cues to meanings that lie under the surface content of their verbalizations (reading between the lines).
*Using value statements and clichés.* These often are perceived as trite and not understanding or not interested in the other person's feelings.
*Using false reassurance or superficial flattery.* This does not make an individual feel better, and is not helpful in establishing open, honest communication.
*Failing to clarify.* Communication is facilitated by clarifying responses. Failing to do so causes multiple interpretations of information.

## The Skill of Listening

Administrators are frequently trained to communicate effectively; however, only a few demonstrate listening to

## Management Spotlight

*Personality conflicts* or *communication* breakdowns are really perception problems.
**Push for high quality communication.**

understand rather than respond. By listening well to the word received, reading manners of expression and body language that is conveyed, leaders can more successfully and proactively direct activities. Managers that react, respond defensively, or respond without complete understanding of what was received, immediately construct an unintentional communication barrier.

The groundwork for effective listening is built around the following As (Rowland, 1994):

**Availability**   Be accessible to staff and colleagues.

**Attentiveness**   Be receptive in the manner in which you listen. Maintain eye contact and positive body language. Reserve judgmental assessment until after communication is delivered. Practice courtesy.

**Acceptance**   Understand the sender's frame of reference. Request clarification if any point is unclear. Guarantee the right of others to speak out. Focus any disagreement on content, not people.

### Communication: Foundation of Team Building

Clear communication is the foundation for team building and maintaining an effective work group. The following steps may assist in communicating more effectively (Rowland & Rowland, 1994):

1. Identify objectives in advance. Plan the mode of communication, expressed content, and targeted receivers.

2. Expressions must be articulated clearly and sometimes rehearsed. Be concise, succinct, and recap the emphasized points.

3. To gain greater acceptance, be mindful to formulate information/communication in a manner that is attuned to the receivers' self-interests. When possible, use relevant analogies.

4. Adjust messages in accordance with the varied personnel skill levels, educational preparation, previous experiences, frames of reference, and differences in needs and cultures.

5. Use conversational language, but be aware that some words have different contexts of meaning. Keep it simple and to the point.

6. Be a skilled listener. Listen to understand, not respond. Elicit criticism and feedback from receivers. Balance negative feedback. Do not accept negative feedback as a personal attack, but instead, accept it as an opportunity to learn. Negative feedback may bear some truth.

7. Provide feedback to subordinates, as well as other organizational stakeholders. Communicate progress reports, as well as results.

8. Use a variety of communication modes to reinforce messages. Initially, use a single most appropriate mode according to the nature of the message. Some messages may be too involved or formal to send out over e-mail, thus warranting personal conversation or a formal meeting.

9. The sender must have credibility. The personal and professional credibility of the information given has been shown to be more important in effecting the desired outcome than the content (Sullivan & Decker, 1989).

10. Information giving is not communication.

11. The responsibility for clarity resides with the sender.

12. Acknowledgment of the contributions of others is essential to foster an atmosphere of cooperation and participant satisfaction.

Communication in any organization can always be improved. Communication barriers occur in various practice settings as a result of varying frames of reference for the receivers. Leaders and managers are challenged to continuously strengthen their personal communication skills, as well as disseminating and receiving accurate information throughout an organization.

Various forms of communication exist; commonly used are e-mail, voice mail, and memorandums. One infrequently used form of management communication is the poem. According to Dr. Ralph Allen (1993), poetry can have a purposeful value in management practice. Dr. Allen further asserts that poems communicate feelings, direction, principle, and message in a qualitative manner. A poem provides managers with an opportunity to communicate a message and demonstrate the caring side of the manager.

The humanist side of management is captured in the following two examples of poems used in the business (Boxes 1-4 and 1-5). Instead of sending a dry note to a licensed staff member to show proof of licensure renewal, a manager could convey the message in an informal and supportive manner.

---

**BOX 1-4**

### ON BEING ON TIME FOR LICENSE/REGISTRATION RENEWING

This is simply a friendly reminder
that noted in your personnel binder
is the fact that your STATE REGISTRATION
expires with your birth celebration.
Surveyors, when finding these little glitches
become hysteric—baring fangs and twitches.
So this little task we'd like you to do—
Please bring us a copy of renewal that's true.
We'll place the proof in your personnel binder
for legal support and a survey that's kinder.

---

From Allen, R. K. (1993). Poetry as a healthcare management tool. *Journal of Poetry Therapy;* 6(4), 229-234.

BOX 1-5

# THOUGHTS ON BEING A NURSE MANAGER

**Ralph Allen**

There is a link in the cement
of health-care's team management
that needs some lifting or more support
as we improve our proud old fort.
The chart displays the chain of command,
visual links from the flag to the sand—
and somewhere twixt top and what shows as the bottom
are two marvelous stars whose commitment has got 'em.
They're known for their patience, their humor and brain
and names they have also; like Kathy and Jane.
Sometimes it appears that they have heavy switches
but feel instead, pureed in sandwiches.
For caught in the middle, pecked at by both layers
of people who act like they're only just players;
some demanding for more out of troops thinly spread,
some asking for milk to help swallow the bread.
    "Consider the budget, manage the sick,
    provide higher quality, make orders stick,
    get more out of this, do more of that,
    the patients are griping, . . . where's Lucy's hat?
    Find all the tasks that were not done today,
    (it will never end, . . . no matter what may);
    tell doctor what's new in room 311,
find chaplain or help, . . . it stinks to high heaven,
these charts are a mess, where are the care plans,
whose turn is it now to clean the bedpans?
Why isn't this done, the State could arrive,
    'Nurse where's my pill . . . I'm hardly alive,
    why must I do this, it's Francis' bed,
    I've got to go home—I'm sick to my head,'
Who messed up the time cards, the treatment's not done,
    (I got into this work 'cause I thought it'd be fun?)
Why is Mom going upstairs, or back down,
Who left her at supper dressed only in gown,
Who can see if Dad's pills are just right,
I'm in a bad mood, so don't pick a fight,
I said I'm not doing that section today,

*Continued*

**BOX 1-5—cont'd**

I've been on vacation since early in May,
My schedule is off and I'm really mad,
and it isn't my fault that the dressing went bad,
there aren't any pads, or blankets to use,
I think you should fix that stupid old fuse,
the call lights don't work, cause she ate the string . . ."
Does any of this have a familiar ring?
Whose duty is it to see that all works?
Who gets to be named as unspeakable jerks?
Who benefits by all the tears and the mis-anger?
Of course, you guessed right—the Sandwiched Nurse Manager.
For all of this joy and all of this fun
is what keeps our nurse managers in flight, on the run.
I think that a look at their place on our chart
should be done by rethinking and not just by art.
The shadow of this, sheds hope and shows care
cause none could be done without your presence there.
You form the point, you take gobs of heat
and go home to soak your tired aching feet.
But please raise the questions and help us to think
of how we can help you skate right on the brink.

---

At the time of publication, Dr. Allen was the President of St. Luke's Extended Care Center. He enjoys acknowledging employees through his poetry. The above effort is in recognition of nurse managers throughout the Empire Health Services system.

## COMMITTEE LEADERSHIP RESPONSIBILITIES

At all levels of management, one is expected to facilitate, chair, or lead meetings. The following guidelines will assure that the meeting is organized, well-planned, and productive (Modified from Stevens, 1989).

I. Preparation of the Physical Environment
   A. Ensure comfort levels by:
      1. Adequate ventilation, light, comfortable room temperature.
      2. Comfortable seating, as well as seating arrangement.
      3. Adequate visual and sound arrangements.

4. Adequate space for writing or referencing material by participant.
5. For longer meetings, it is nice to have ice water available.

B. Ensure participant convenience by:
1. Supply extra paper, pencils, etc. as needed.
2. Minimize interruptions:
   a. Inform operator of who is in the meeting and who will take messages.
   b. Request that audio be turned off on pagers and that cellulars not be used during meeting. (*Many participants already acknowledge this as professional courtesy.*)
   c. Mark all entry doors to signify what meeting is in progress.
3. Prepare and check out all necessary audiovisual aids to be used in presentations.
4. Supply agendas and documents to be discussed. (Do not assume that everyone will remember to bring the original copy.)

II. Preparation of Participants
A. Send a reminder before the meeting date (i.e., memo, e-mail, voice-mail).
B. Distribute detailed agendas far enough in advance for necessary preparation or research of topics to be discussed.
C. Distribute for advance preparation any documents to be approved or analyzed.
D. Indicate any materials that the participant should bring to the meeting.
E. Prepare any participants that are anticipated to present on new or follow-up topics.

III. Leader Preparation
A. Prepare an agenda that clearly indicates the purpose and content of the meeting.
B. Review the status of all agenda topics to date.
C. Gather all necessary background information and supportive data on agenda topics.

    D. Determine who needs to be invited as resource persons based on agenda topics. (To maximize productivity, determine in advance which participants should be invited based on agenda topic, individuals' expertise, and expected contribution to the meeting.)

    E. Prepare a list of critical questions that can stimulate committee interaction on agenda topics.

    F. Prepare such handouts or audiovisual presentations that will facilitate committee understanding of topics.

    G. Prepare a strategy or strategies for conducting the meeting.

    H. Determine who will take minutes/record-keeping.

IV. End of Meeting Preparation

    A. Leader's responsibility to summarize what has occurred during the committee interactions.

    B. Identify the decisions reached.

    C. Summarize objective for next meeting if needed; set date and time for next meeting if appropriate.

    D. Summarize homework directions and specific assignments if necessary.

    E. Ensure minutes are prepared.

## COMMITTEES

Every committee should have a purpose and precise responsibility. Members should be selected according to their unique contributions. Each plays a vital role in achieving the work of the group. Committees should be of manageable size for discussion and disagreement. The group leader should have a working knowledge of group dynamics to facilitate the committee's effectiveness. Swansburg (1990) asserts the following standards for evaluation of nursing committees:

- The committee has been established by appropriate authority: by laws, executive appointment, or other.
- There are a stated purpose, objectives, and operational procedures for the committee.

- There is a mechanism for consultation between chairs and persons to whom they report.
- There is a published agenda for each committee meeting.
- Committee members are surveyed beforehand to obtain agenda items including problems, plans, and sharing of news.
- There is an effective chair for each committee.
- Recorded minutes of each committee are used to evaluate its effectiveness in meeting stated objectives.
- Committee membership is manageable and representative of the expertise needed and the people they affect.
- Nurses are adequately represented on all appropriate institutional committees.

### Advantages of Committees

Committees are participatory group processes. Committees are designed to (Swansburg, 1991):
- Be effective in group problem-solving.
- Be effective within larger organization, as well as within the division or unit of nursing. Sometimes this is expanded to include appropriate professional organizations, institutions of higher learning, and ancillary departments.
- Achieve legitimacy.
- Acquire resources and approval for their ideas.
- Motivate others in the organization to accept, implement, and support their new group solution.

### Bylaws

In establishing bylaws, the committee must have them approved through the appropriate administrative channels and the appropriate physician staff committee. The following components (articles) are essential components of bylaws:

|  |  |
|---|---|
| Article I | Name |
| Article II | Purpose and Function |
| Article III | Members |

## TIME MANAGEMENT AND PRIORITY SETTING

Time management tips that can indeed make a difference are listed in the *Action Tips* box. However, there are time management seminars and personal development programs available should this be an area for individual development.

## Action Tips

### TIME MANAGEMENT

- Make and use "to do" lists or planners when possible.
- Give total attention to each task.
- Complete each task the first time when possible.
- Be considerate of other people's time.
- Minimize meetings (use only if other means of communication are not appropriate).
- Use telephone time-savers (i.e., outline basic points before call; determine a time allotment to be on the phone).
- Eliminate unproductive reading (read reports and other documents once and act or reply at once; read less essential material on a break or while traveling).
- Close the door when there are jobs that must be completed (successful control of interruptions is essential).
- Follow up at the end of the day (analyze what tasks were not completed; track and eliminate time-killers; give them top priority the next day).
- Eliminate paper (do not allow it to accumulate).
- Conduct regularly scheduled staff meetings.

## Action Tips —cont'd

### *TIME MANAGEMENT—cont'd*

- Block your time (involves planning).
- Take time to train colleagues and subordinates (saves time and increases productivity; ties in with delegation).
- Relinquish ownership of problems that are not yours to solve (involving employees in problem solving at point of service when possible).
- Learn the fine art of saying no (refuse to accept tasks that you cannot do at the time).
- Plan emergencies (expect the unexpected and marginal emergencies can be controlled).
- Plan minivacations daily. (Briefly get away from the work related activity during the day: eat lunch outside; take a brisk walk around the parking lot; listen to music, etc.).
- Pick a regularly scheduled day to completely clear your desk and totally reprioritizing projects.
- Check off tasks as completed—it does feel great!

Modified from Rowland, H., & Rowland, B. (1995). *Nursing administration manual* (vols. 1-2). Rockville, MD: Aspen Publishers; and Marelli, T. (1997). *The nurse manager's survival guide.* St. Louis: Mosby.

**Leadership**

### Assigning Priorities

In planning activities to achieve maximum results, you must plan to be effective, not just efficient. Planning answers four basic questions: Where am I now? *(Assess)* Where do I need/want to be? *(Goal)* How do I achieve this? *(Plan)* When do I anticipate yielding results? *(Implementation/Evaluation)*.

In planning, one must set priorities (group tasks into categories).

| | |
|---|---|
| High Priority: | Most important; handle at once. |
| Mid Priority: | Less urgent; do when you get to it. |
| Low Priority: | Low priority; keep it just in case or toss. |

## Delegation

### *Degrees of Delegation*

Delegating can be assigned in the following ways (Baille, 1989):

1. Asking the person to make the decision or take action without the need to give you feedback.
2. Asking the person to take action but to let you know what was done.
3. Asking the person to take action only in part and to confer with you before taking further action.
4. Asking that the person not take action but report to you with an analysis of all possible alternatives.
5. Asking the person to explore a problem and report to you the facts necessary for making an informed decision.

### *Guidelines For Effective Delegation*

Delegating effectively saves time, increases productivity, and subsequently challenges and enhances the professional growth of individuals in any job assignment or clinical setting (Data from Rowland, 1994; Sullivan & Decker, 1998).

- State the plan and identify the task clearly.
- Allow sufficient time to do the task.
- Select the person for the assignment carefully and know why that person was selected.
- Ensure that communication strategies are kept open.
- Develop feedback and reporting mechanisms as necessary.
- Inspect what you expect; however, do not micromanage.
- Hold the employee accountable and stay in control.
- Initially, consider delegating tasks that you do best.
- Complete a time analysis; choose activities on which you regularly spend a significant amount of time.
- Consider delegating one of those activities per week.
- Build self-confidence by rewarding those who do the job well and demonstrate initiative and commitment to the department.
- Always give people the tools needed to complete a task.

*Steps In the Delegation Process*

Delegation is sharing responsibility and authority with subordinates and holding them accountable for performance. At every level, the supervisor is accountable for the successes and failures of subordinates (Sullivan & Decker, 1989).

1. Identify areas where delegation is appropriate.
2. Plan before delegating.
3. Define the responsibility to be assigned in terms of delegated objectives and the specific results to be achieved.
4. Determine the tools and resources that are available to achieve expected results and identify the appropriate limitations.
5. Make the assignment effectively, building in provisions for established deadlines and progress reports.
6. Demonstrate ongoing support of project or task that was delegated.

## MANAGING CHANGE

Planned change is a thoughtful and purposeful effort that is carefully managed to improve systems or create a positive outcome (Box 1-6). There are many change theorists and models cited as classics in the management literature. Each person has adopted a favorite that is utilized more often than others. However, the nursing process also serves as a basis for problem solving.

## High Performers Lead the Charge

The reengineering and redesign of healthcare organizational processes and jobs is gaining widespread acceptance as organizations intensify efforts to provide high quality, cost-effective care in the midst of increased competition and regulatory reforms. According to the Hay Hospital Compensation Survey, more than half of the institutions surveyed were actively involved in work redesign and many have completed such initiatives.

**BOX 1-6**

## AN ECLECTIC APPROACH: THE NURSING PROCESS

| Nursing Process | Change Process |
|---|---|
| Assessment | 1. Identify the problem or opportunity |
| | 2. Collect data |
| | 3. Analyze data |
| Planning | 4. Plan the change strategies |
| Implementation | 5. Implement the change |
| Evaluation | 6. Evaluate effectiveness |
| | 7. Stabilize the change |

From Sullivan, E., & Decker, P. (1998). *Effective management in nursing.* Menlo Park, CA: Addison-Wesley Publishing.

A separate Hay study on organizational effectiveness and productivity, reported that high performing successful hospitals do the following (Pierson & Williams, 1995):

- Adopt strategies to gain and sustain dominance, as well as nurture physician and managed care partnerships.
- Develop more streamlined organizational structures and management processes that are better aligned with those institutions' business strategies and markets.
- Create stronger, more positive cultures that focus on clarity of direction, decision making, and performance.
- Redesign human resources functions to be more closely linked to the business strategy and organization work culture, and that emphasize role clarity, performance, team building, and flexibility.
- Continue to reduce layers of managers.
- Emphasize cross-functional processes rather than traditional departmental specialties.

The survey found that these high performing organizations also have lower relative costs and higher productivity in line management and key staff functions. Needless to say, effective communication is paramount in successful implementation of these strategies.

---

**BOX 1-7**

## MYTHS AND REALITIES OF ORGANIZATIONAL CHANGE

| Myth | Reality |
|------|---------|
| This will go away. | Change is here to stay. |
| It will help if I get upset about this. | Controlling emotions increases control over the situation. |
| This is a bad thing for my career. | Progress often masquerades as trouble. |
| I can just keep on doing my job like I have been. | If the company or organization is changing, you probably need to be changing, too. |
| All these problems prove that the changes are bad for the company. | Problems are a natural side effect of the change process. |
| Top management knows a lot more than they are telling. | The odds are that management is being as open and straightforward as the situations permit. |
| Management doesn't care about people. | Management has to make some tough decisions, and it's impossible to keep everyone happy. |
| I am not in a position to make a difference. | You are either part of the solution or part of the problem. |
| Top management is supposed to make the changes work. | If you work here, this is your plan. |

From Pritchett, P., & Pound, R. (1994). *Employee handbook for organizational change.* Dallas: Pritchett Associates.

## Implementing and Supporting Organizational Change

When organizational changes occur, people frequently develop a negative mind set based on misinterpretation, faulty assumptions, ill motives, and inaccurate perceptions. Unnecessary problems are encountered unless the misperceptions or "myths" are challenged (Pritchett & Pound, 1994) (Box 1-7).

## Review of Change Theories

Most healthcare providers that have a baccalaureate degree grew up on change theories as part of the foundation for leadership and management instruction. The most widely cited in the literature today, are the same: Reddin, Lewin, Rogers, Havelock, and Lippitt. With any change, regardless of magnitude, communication is essential to the success of the change. Swansburg (1991) lists four announcements that should be made by management for optimum success:

- That a change will be made.
- What the decision is and why it was made.
- How the decision will be implemented.
- How the implementation is progressing.

**Reddin** asserts seven techniques by which change can be accomplished (Swansburg, 1991):

1. Diagnosis
2. Mutual setting of objectives
3. Group emphasis
4. Maximum information
5. Discussion of implementation
6. Use of ceremony and ritual
7. Resistance interpretation

**Lewin's** theory involves three stages:

1. *The unfreezing stage*  This stage occurs when disequilibrium is introduced, the problem identified, creating a need for change. The nurse manager diagnoses the problem (scientific problem solving with projected probable outcomes) and best solution selected.
2. *The moving stage*  The nurse manager gathers information and a detailed action plan is made. Trial runs are sometimes done; other times the change is simply implemented.
3. *The refreezing stage*  Changes are integrated and stabilized into the organization. Outcomes are monitored; continuous performance improvement.

**Roger's** theory is a modification from Lewin's theory. There are five phases:

| | | |
|---|---|---|
| Phase 1: | Awareness | (corresponds to the unfreezing stage of Lewin) |
| Phase 2: | Interest | (corresponds |
| Phase 3: | Evaluation | to |
| Phase 4: | Trial | moving phase) |
| Phase 5: | Adoption | (corresponds to Lewin's refreezing stage) |

Roger's theory depends on five factors for success (Swansburg, 1991):

- The change must have the relative advantage of being better than existing methods.
- It must be compatible with existing values.
- Complexity—more complex ideas persist even though simple ones are implemented more easily.
- Divisibility—change is introduced on a small scale.
- Communicability—the easier the change is to describe, the more likely it is to spread.

**Havelock's** theory is another rendition of Lewin's theory. Havelock expanded to six elements (the first three correspond to unfreezing, the next two to moving, and the last) to unfreezing. Havelock emphasizes planning as being the significant element for success.

1. Building a relationship
2. Diagnosis
3. Acquiring relevant resources
4. Choosing a solution
5. Gaining acceptance
6. Stabilization and self-renewal

**Lippett's** theory added a seventh element to Lewin's theory. The seven phases (Swansburg, 1991):

| | |
|---|---|
| Phase 1: | Diagnosing the problem |
| Phase 2: | Assessment of the motivation and capacity for change |

Phase 3:    Assessment of the change agent's motivation
            and resources
Phase 4:    Selecting progressive change objectives
Phase 5:    Choosing the appropriate role for the change agent
Phase 6:    Maintenance of the change
Phase 7:    Termination of the helping relationship (the change
            agent withdraws after policy implemented)

## Strategies for Overcoming Obstacles to Change

Attempting to maintain the status quo when efforts are initiated to alter it, is a common response to change. Change can be stressful, which subsequently evokes resistance. Factors that stimulate resistance to change include individual stress levels, habits, complacency, fear, perceived loss of power, perceived increase in workload, ego involvement, insecurity, perceived loss of relationships, and loss of rewards. Swansburg (1991) published nine strategies for overcoming obstacles to change:

1. *Managing Change*  Change can be viewed as opportunities, challenging, and refreshing. Effective management is dependent on the nurse leader and his or her effectiveness as a change agent.

2. *Collection and Development of Data*  Nurse leaders must have useful information. The data must be discussed, analyzed, and utilized to effect change during implementation, but also used to monitor performance after implementation.

3. *Preparation of Planning*  Preplanning helps managers match the right people with the right tasks. It is also helpful in keeping interpersonal relationships from disruption. Planning helps minimize anxiety produced with change. For change to be optimally successful for patient care services, it is this author's belief that it is imperative that the nurse executive and nurse managers be involved in some components of the strategic planning process.

4. *Training and Education*  The frequency of training and education should match the frequency and magnitude of

change. It is a challenge to determine the triggers to stimulate desired learning; however, people need to comprehend the change that is affecting them.

5. *Rewards*   Rewards for old behavior patterns should be removed after change has been proposed. Compensation programs are not always feasible; however, other rewards can be implemented: communication of standards of practice, performance evaluations, special certificates and ceremonies, job enrichment, and encouraging self-development.

6. *Groups as Change Agents*   When groups work in harmony and share the same vision and goals, change is effective. The informal groups can promote and support change. Often, the organization's informal leaders champion initiatives with less resistance than management.

7. *Communications*   Announcements are factual and comprehensive. Any blanks will be filled in by rumors and speculations, thus producing more anxiety. Managers should also address projected obstacles to resistance and reasons for resistance in the communication. This makes individuals aware of and accountable for their own behavior in response to change.

8. *The Organizational Environment*   Managers need to be committed to change and support it with their own actions and attitudes. Managers can establish a healthy environment by:
   - Stressing relationships with each other
   - Emphasizing mutual trust and confidence
   - Emphasizing interdependence and sharing responsibility; promoting can-do attitudes
   - Containing group membership and responsibility by limiting individuals from belonging to too many groups
   - Sharing control and responsibility
   - Resolving conflict immediately.

9. *Anticipating Potential Failures*   Determine risks involved, resources required, who best to do the job. Plan a flexible agenda and action plan so that when mistakes do happen, one can still move forward.

Managers create the environment that fosters and encourages new ideas that can facilitate change. Creativity is original thought and action as an expression to a challenge. Innovation is the ability to put new ideas into operation. To manage change, leaders need to develop creative problem solving skills. Lattimer and Winitsky (Swansburg, 1991) suggest the following as one strategy for creative problem solving. More detailed problem solving techniques are discussed in Chapter 3.

*Thinking* Identify factors related to solving the issue or developing a plan of action. Make the choice between related levels of risk of selected alternatives.

*Decomposing* Break down the situation into smaller components: issues, alternatives, uncertainties, consequences. Work through each to facilitate decision.

*Simplifying* Make intuitive judgments on the crucial factors and most essential relationships.

*Specifying* Establish values and structure for key factors and projected outcomes.

*Rethinking* Review the original analysis for rationale, omissions, and priorities.

With any problem solving model used, reliability and validation of solutions must be incorporated in the process. Drucker (1985) asserts that every organization needs a strategy for innovation. He suggests the following strategies for innovation:

1. *The first with the mostest.* Discourage competitors by being the first in the market for a new or improved service or product that is value-oriented.
2. *The second with the mostest* Let someone else establish the market, but offer few features and specified capabilities (e.g., drug-dependency facility).
3. *The niche strategy* Corner a finite market, making it not feasible or not profitable for others.
4. *Making the product your carrier* One product carries another (e.g., a medication cart with several optional features that are priced separately).

## Becoming a Change Agent

1. *Control Your Attitude*   Become a change agent by concentrating energies on becoming a champion of initiatives that are congruent with the new directions of the organization. Seize organizational changes as opportunities to learn and grow. Choose deliberately to be optimistic, enthusiastic, and energetic. You will benefit far more than the organization will.

2. *Take Some Ownership of the Changes*   Complaining is not the same as contributing. Identify problems or opportunities, but then have the guts to suggest and commit to workable solutions. The best way to protect your job is to become flexible, adaptable, and marketable.

3. *Choose Your Battles Carefully*   Your reputation is your most valuable asset. Do not fight losing battles. It is easier to ride the wind than run against it: Concentrate on keeping the wind to your back.

4. *Be Tolerant of Mistakes*   What looks like a mistake may be precisely the right move; or the best move under the circumstances. Many times when choosing a lesser evil, there are trade-offs involved.

5. *Keep Your Sense of Humor*   Crying is cleansing, but humor is healing. An upbeat attitude will not keep you from stressful situations, but will help you handle the stressful situations.

6. *Do not Let Your Strengths Become Weaknesses*   Shift your job's priorities to match the changes in organizational priorities. Align yourself with any changes in values and corporate culture. Develop new competencies. Be alert; catch on; refocus rapidly. Continuing to focus on *doing what you do best* might be one of the worst things you could do.

7. *Practice Good Stress Management Techniques*   Adjusting to new circumstances causes emotional labor; therefore practice tension releasing strategies such as vigorous physical activity.

8. *Support Top Management*   Top management desperately needs support. It is hard to be a hero during peace time; however, amidst major change, there are opportunities to lead the organization.

9. *Invent the Future Instead of Trying to Redesign the Past* The best way to predict the future is to put yourself in charge of creating the situation that you want. Be purposeful, benchmark against *best practices*, and take action toward implementing that vision. Take cues from the external environment and proactively focus on new directions (Pritchett & Pound, 1994).

Action tips are miscellaneous quips and quotes collected over the years that are fun to use when developing others (*Action Tips* box). Moreover, each one carries a powerful message.

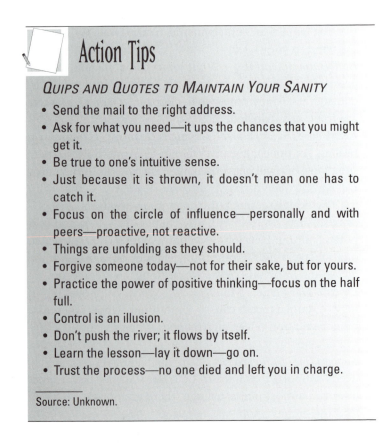

# Action Tips

## QUIPS AND QUOTES TO MAINTAIN YOUR SANITY

- Send the mail to the right address.
- Ask for what you need—it ups the chances that you might get it.
- Be true to one's intuitive sense.
- Just because it is thrown, it doesn't mean one has to catch it.
- Focus on the circle of influence—personally and with peers—proactive, not reactive.
- Things are unfolding as they should.
- Forgive someone today—not for their sake, but for yours.
- Practice the power of positive thinking—focus on the half full.
- Control is an illusion.
- Don't push the river; it flows by itself.
- Learn the lesson—lay it down—go on.
- Trust the process—no one died and left you in charge.

Source: Unknown.

## THE LEADER AS A TEAM BUILDER

Most decisions are made in teams; so team learning is essential for successful learning organizations (Boxes 1-8 and 1-9). Gauthier (1996) published that successful, learning teams:

- Share a Vision: Clear definition of the desired outcomes.
- Hold themselves accountable for high performance.
- Live by behavioral ground rules.
- Have a high level of trust among teammates.

---

**BOX 1-8**

### CHARACTERISTICS OF EFFECTIVE TEAMS

**An effective team:**

- is not limited to a departmental work group. Its members have greater multidirectional communication. Include vendors, customers, people from other departments, and key staff personnel.
- possesses all the necessary knowledge, skill, and experience required to get the job done.
- searches for excellence in quality, productivity, and customer service. It removes factors that inhibit quality performance.
- welcomes innovation, new services, and new techniques is willing to take risks.
- is democratic. There is an absence of rank or formal authority. Leaders refer to his/her own co-workers as associates or colleagues.
- adheres to ethical and moral considerations.
- Demonstrates openness and candor. Is inspired by a vision of what it is trying to accomplish. Its goals are clear and all are working toward same goals.
- actively constructs formal and informal networks.
- has power that is based not on formal authority but on the team's credibility.
- has members who trust each other and are sensitive to each other's needs. They understand roles and responsibilities.
- minimizes conflict with other teams or other nonteam members through collaboration, cooperation.
- is optimistic and has fun.

---

From Umiker, W. (1994). Management skills for the new health care supervisor. In Rowland, H., & Rowland, B. (Eds.). (1995). *Nursing administration manual*. Rockville, MD: Aspen Publishers.

- Reason productively about members' behavior and team dynamics.
- Challenge one another's positions openly.
- Acknowledge and avoid defensive reasoning.
- Learn from mistakes and failures.

---

**BOX 1-9**

## MARRIOT LEADERSHIP PLEDGE

TO: Myself
SUBJECT: A Pledge for (year): A Rededication to Excellence in Leadership

*I promise the members of my team:*

1. To set the right example for them by my own actions in all things.
2. To be consistent in my temperament so that they know how to "read" me and what to expect from me.
3. To be fair, impartial, and consistent in matters relating to work rules, discipline, and rewards.
4. To show sincere, personal interest in them as individuals without becoming overly familiar.
5. To seek their counsel on matters that affect their jobs and to be guided as much as possible by their judgement.
6. To allow them as much individuality as possible in the way their jobs are performed, as long as the quality of the end result is not compromised.
7. To make sure they always know in advance what I expect from them in the way of conduct and performance on the job.
8. To be appreciative of their efforts and generous in praise of their accomplishments.
9. To use every opportunity to teach them how to do their jobs better and how to help themselves advance in skill level and responsibility.
10. To show them that I can "do," as well as "manage," by pitching in to work beside them when my help is needed.

Signed:_____

---

From Batten, J. (1989). *Tough-minded leadership.* New York: AMACOM (American Management Association).

## Bibliography

Allen, R.K. (1993). Poetry as a healthcare management tool. *Journal of Poetry Therapy,* 6(4), 229-234.

Baille, V., & Cordoni, T. (1989). Effective nursing. In H. Rowland & B. Rowland (Eds.), *Nursing administration manual.* Rockville, MD: Aspen Publishers.

Batten, J. (1989). *Tough-minded leadership.* New York: AMACOM (American Management Association).

Chitty, K. (1993). *Professional nursing: Concepts & challenges.* Philadelphia: WB Saunders.

Drucker, P. (1995). *Managing in a time of change.* New York: Truman Tally Books/Dutton.

Drucker, P. (1985). Creating strategies of innovation. *Planning Review,* November, 8-11, 45.

Gauthier, A. (1996). Systems thinking helps leaders handle change. *Health Progress,* Jan/Feb, 44-45.

Longest, B. (1998). Managerial competence at senior levels of integrated delivery systems. *Journal of Healthcare Management,* 43(2), 115-133.

Marelli, T. (1997). *The nurse manager's survival guide.* St. Louis: Mosby.

Pierson, D., & Williams, J. (1994). Compensation via integration. *Hospital & Health Networks,* Sept 5, 28-38.

Pritchett, P. (1997). *The team member handbook for teamwork.* Dallas: Pritchett & Associates.

Pritchett, P., & Pound, R. (1994). *Employee handbook for organizational change.* Dallas: Pritchett & Associates.

Rowland, H., & Rowland, B. (1995). *Volume 1: Nursing administration manual.* Rockville, MD: Aspen Publishers.

Rowland, H., & Rowland, B. (1995). *Volume 2: Nursing administration manual.* Rockville, MD: Aspen Publishers.

Secretan, L. (1997). *Reclaiming higher ground.* Alton, Ontario: Macmillan Canada Publishing.

Senge, P. (1994). *The fifth discipline fieldbook.* New York: Bantam Doubleday Dell Publishing.

Spitzer-Lehman, R. (1989). Middle management consolidation. Nursing Management, 20(8). In H. Rowland & B. Rowland (Eds.). *Nursing administration manual.* Rockville, MD: Aspen Publishers.

Starkweather, D., & Shropshire, D. (1994). Management effectiveness. Manual of Health Services Management, R. Taylor (ed.). In H. Rowland & B. Rowland, (Eds.). *Nursing administration manual.* Rockville, MD: Aspen Publishers.

Stevens, B. (1989). *The nurse executive.* Rockville, MD: Aspen Publisher.

Sullivan, E., & Decker, P. (1989). *Effective management in nursing.* Menlo Park, CA: Addison-Wesley Publishing.

Swansburg, R. (1990). *Management and leadership for nurse managers.* Boston: Jones and Bartlett Publishers.

Umiker, W. (1981). Decision making and problem solving by the busy professional. Healthcare Supervisor, 7(4). In H. Rowland & B. Rowland (Eds.). *Nursing administration manual* (1995). Rockville, MD: Aspen Publishers.

Wolford, G., Maeller, D., & Johnson, K. (1992). Bridging the leadership gap. *Healthcare Forum Journal,* 35(3): 19-27.

# Chapter 2

# Human Resource Principles

## The Hiring Process

C. Daniel Gorman and Sandra Pierson

---

*Experience is not what happens to you. It is what you do with what happens to you.*

*Aldous Huxley*

What does the nurse manager need to know in the realm of human resources and why? This subject brings consternation for the most able of managers in all endeavors, not just in nursing. Making consistently good personnel decisions is extremely important. Everything is at stake: time, money, the manager's sanity, the prospective employee's welfare, the team's welfare, the patient's welfare, and, last but not least, overall customer satisfaction. Every aspect of the nurse manager's job is strongly impacted by personnel decisions. Failure to make appropriate decisions regarding personnel can undermine all the efforts put forth in managing the unit.

There is no way to run a unit without people—the correct people. Herein lies the first daunting task that faces the nurse manager.

What kind of and how many people do I need? Is the skill mix correct to accomplish all necessary patient care? Are the position descriptions up-to-date and correct? Do they reflect the latest levels in skills, equipment, license requirements, certification, and competency? Is the mission statement of

**50**

**Management Spotlight**

- Effective team players help drive discipline into the group.
- High performance team players police themselves!
- High performers hold themselves, and each other, accountable for top notch results.

From Pritchett, P. (1997). *The team member handbook for teamwork.* Dallas: Pritchett & Associates.

the unit current? Does it fit in the grand scheme of the facility? Are the functions of the unit current and complete? Does the authorized staffing match the functional requirements? If the answer to these questions is "yes," then the nurse manager is ready to proceed with staffing the unit.

## POSITION DESCRIPTIONS

A nurse manager must stay current with position control. The position control report specifies the present allowance of full-time equivalents (FTEs): full-time employees (FTs), part-time employees, and PRN (pro renata) (PKs) as the occasion requires. Position descriptions should be on file for every *different* position in the unit. They are the building blocks that the successful manager uses for candidate selection, training and development, performance appraisal, compensation, and organizational structure.

It is recommended that position descriptions be general. Every possible task does not need to be listed. The position should be outlined, and the dimensions or scope should be spelled out in brief terms. Each employee should be able to remember all the tasks in his or her position description. There should be no confusion in the employee's mind about what is expected. When it becomes necessary to update a position description, the manager must remember to review and revise the following:

- Selection criteria
- Training and development plan
- Performance appraisal
- Compensation
- Organizational structure

All these personnel-related actions must be done in concert with the human resources staff. They in turn will coordinate with other departments, such as finance and corporate legal, before any recommended changes can become fact. For the new manager there are many facets to personnel that make this topic a minefield. Be patient and follow the corporate guidelines. Although they may seem bothersome at first, in the final analysis they often are the best and only way to accomplish change.

## RECRUITING

The job search and the process of filling a position have many similarities. For ease of discussion, these similarities will be addressed as follows:

- Networking
- Advertising
- Agencies
- Cold Call

### Networking

Networking allows friends, acquaintances, and professional colleagues to help you in filling a position. It requires personal contact and a willingness to spend the time and effort necessary to make those who might know of a lead (almost anyone) aware of your needs. Obviously, people cannot help you with your search unless they know your requirements. The key to success is to make your initial contacts and then to stay in touch with them. They may know of a person who is looking for a position just like the one you're trying to fill.

Several considerations come into play in networking. The first is the immediate opportunity to question the person providing the name of the potential employee. The more detailed and honest this exchange is, the easier it will be to decide whether or not to call the suggested/recommended person. Frequent contact with the network chain is important because new "leads" may become available on a daily or weekly basis. This approach requires persistence, not a wait-and-see attitude.

As a networking manager, you can establish credibility with your networking chain by returning the favor for colleagues who are also in need of qualified candidates. Once you become known as a manager who needs certain types of personnel or knows of opportunities for certain personnel, a natural dialogue will develop. As with all managerial tasks, networking takes time and the ability to manage information exchange effectively.

The school circuit is often a good network. Keep your former classmates, professors, and others, such as the college placement personnel, in the loop. You never know where the "right" candidate will be uncovered.

The key to success in networking is that you stay in charge. The search is your responsibility. Let contacts know that you will be calling them again and when: "Would 11:00 tomorrow morning be good?" To prompt yourself to make those calls, remember all the times you have been told, "Oh, I meant to tell you. . . ."

**Human Resource Principles**

### Advertising

Advertising is all-important in attracting the right candidates to your position. If the department position descriptions are well done, one of the first hurdles has been overcome. Recruiting can be difficult in rural areas and in some of the large metropolitan areas. How do you attract attention to your advertisement? What do you offer in the way of educational and other benefits to overcome the objections? (Caution: Do not offer something that will not materialize.)

As with any written material, clarity and brevity are paramount. On the other hand, specific needs and requirements must be clearly stated to avoid confusion. Applicants who do not fit the bill are wasting their time and yours. Where will this ad appear? Once the ad has cleared human resources (most organizations require this step), what are the most effective venues for the best return?

*Internal recruiting* is the least expensive way to advertise. This morale-boosting method has lots of side benefits, ranging from low cost to "knowing the candidate." *Bulletin boards* are effective and inexpensive. Once the notice has been posted, the networking starts—both internally and externally. An obvious drawback is that the organization could end up with a number of disappointed employees if the ad is not accurate and specific about what is required.

*Local newspapers* are fairly cost-effective if the reading population contains the types of employees being sought. This is difficult to gauge in smaller metropolitan centers, so it is almost a requirement to at least try the local paper. The newspaper's advertising department can provide you with figures on readership and geographic coverage. An added benefit is that larger papers often publish a special want ad supplement that is sold relatively inexpensively.

*Want ads on the web* offer additional exposure and expand the geographic area considerably. The web also provides other options. Several sites allow you to post jobs for a fee, while enticing candidates to job search by scanning the site. Another option is to have your own company web site. Because web sites are multifaceted, many larger organizations have chosen to go the corporate site route. For a smaller company, the key to having your site visited is to have your company name mentioned on as many "links" as possible. The following are sample web sites that offer various services:

1. Online Career Center: www.occ.com
2. Monster Board: www.monster.com
3. America's Job Bank: www.ajb.dni.us

Keep in mind that searching the web for resumés is another way of finding personnel; however, such a search can be time-consuming.

*Professional journals* are another means of broadcasting your needs. In fact, they are a must for hard-to-recruit positions or high-level professional positions. Ads must be sent weeks or months before publication. Pricing is comparable to that of agencies; however, the return gain is usually worth the price.

If a significant dollar commitment is being made, consider an eye-catching display ad. First, grab the reader's attention; continue with more interesting detail; then make sure the contact information is "loud and clear." Several regional areas and states have magazines promoting their attractions. Because promotion is the keynote of these publications, there are advantages to advertising for higher, difficult-to-fill positions in this medium.

Cultural attractions may be a factor in convincing a person to relocate. According to recent surveys done in the top 1000 corporations, reluctance to relocate is increasing. The most frequently noted reason is the lack of permanence in corporate positions and fear of being without a job in a city where the person has no support group. (This is why spouse search is so important to couples when both members need or want to work.)

In responding to an ad, the applicant may refer to seeing your ad in the *National Ad Search*. This weekly folio-style newspaper gathers ads from 75 Sunday papers nationwide and publishes them in an alphabetized and paginated format the following Tuesday. The subscriber pays the cost. This paper is also available on the web for a fee.

## Agencies

A complete discussion of agencies needs to include conventional and contingency recruiters as well as employment agencies, both permanent and temporary. First, however, it is necessary to clarify some potentially confusing differences in dealing with agencies. Firms in the category of "conventional" or "retained" recruiter are retained by the hiring company and are paid a portion of their fee immediately to initiate the search. Occasionally, these firms accept contingency assignments. "Contingency" recruiters and other firms in executive recruiting operate on a fee-paid-on-placement basis. Therefore three or four of these firms might be attempting to fill the same position simultaneously. The only firm that makes any money is the one that actually places the candidate. This situation can cause potential problems for all concerned because candidates may register with numerous agencies. Agencies will unknowingly submit candidates who are also being submitted by another recruiter. Several individual recruiters have excellent working arrangements with companies. Some are former employees of the company who often know the ins and outs of the organization and provide only high-quality candidates.

In today's rush to cut overhead, some companies are outsourcing the recruiting function. A good recruiter can save the company a lot of effort and money. However, a recruiter who provides a poor candidate on even one or two occasions is likely to be dropped from the company's list of acceptable contractors.

Fees paid to recruiters can vary widely, depending on the specialty, the availability of qualified candidates, and the amount of work that goes into obtaining a suitable slate of candidates. A fee based on 15% to 35% of the employee's first-year salary plus a percentage of any bonus is typical. Because some recruiters specialize in certain types of jobs or specific industries, they can be especially helpful in candidate selection.

Employment agencies are a useful resource. Many companies today seldom hire permanent employees as a first step. The temporary-to-permanent employee has become the preferred route. One benefit to the employer is the long observation period, which offers the opportunity to see if the individual has the requisite skills and is trainable without making the commitment to a full-time position. Another is avoidance of the termination process if the employee is not suitable. Temporary employment agencies formulate a working arrangement with the hiring company. If the individual placed at the company in a temporary position is offered and accepts full-time employment, the hiring company pays a finder's fee to the agency instead of the larger fee that would be paid for a regular placement. Another option is that the temporary agency will provide the organization with personnel who work in varying time degrees—from "on call" to a fairly regular schedule. The obvious benefits are the flexibility for both the company and the individual.

### Cold Call

In sales terms the "cold call" is the most difficult of approaches. It involves contacting a person without any introductory preliminaries. The result is that you are talking to a complete stranger who may or may not be qualified for the position. The success statistics for this approach to job seeking are in the single digits, so you can imagine what the success ratio is in job filling! Making cold calls is difficult, time-consuming, and best left to professional recruiters, who have credibility in this approach.

### REVIEWING RESUMÉS AND APPLICATIONS

Wading through applications and resumés can be a tough job. The most helpful aid in reviewing a resumé is a checklist that summarizes the position requirements, taken directly from the position description. Once the checklist is completed, you should have a fair idea about the candidate's ability to fit into your organization. However, there are three "fits"—mission, function, and personality.

Attention to the applicant's resumé is important. For example, be sensitive to the wording of the resume (Box 2-1). There is a great difference between "attended University of New Mexico" and "B.S. in Nursing, University of New Mexico." What action words are used? "Participated in" is not nearly as strong as "led," "developed," "implemented" and "wrote." Is there evidence of accomplishments, or is the resume just a list of duties performed? Has the individual won or been nominated for an award? Certain awards have credibility within an industry, and receiving such an award, or even being nominated, is a fairly good indication of the person's value in his or her last position.

**BOX 2-1**

## ABBREVIATIONS APPEARING ON NURSES' RESUMÉS AND APPLICATIONS

**ANP**   Adult Nurse Practitioner
**CAPA**   Certified Ambulatory Post-Anesthesia Nurse
**CARN**   Certified Addiction Registered Nurse
**CCCN**   Certified Continence Care Nurse
**CCM**   Certified Case Manager
**CCRN**   Certified Critical Care Registered Nurse
**CDE**   Certified Diabetes Educator
**CEN**   Certified Emergency Nurse
**CETN**   Certified Enterostomal Therapy Nurse
**CFRN**   Certified Flight Registered Nurse
**CGRN**   Certified Gastroenterology Registered Nurse
**CHN**   Certified Hemodialysis Nurse
**CIC**   Certified Infection Control
**CNDLTC**   Certified Nurse Director of Long-Term Care
**CNM**   Certified Nurse Midwife
**CNN**   Certified Nephrology Nurse
**CNNP**   Certified Neonatal Nurse Practitioner
**CNOR**   Certified Nurse Operating Room
**CNRN**   Certified Neuroscience Registered Nurse
**CNS**   Clinical Nurse Specialist
**CNSN**   Certified Nutrition Support Nurse
**COCN**   Certified Ostomy Care Nurse
**COHN**   Certified Occupational Health Nurse
**CORLN**   Certified Otorhinolaryngology and Head/Neck Nurse
**CPAN**   Certified Post-Anesthesia Nurse
**CPDN**   Certified Peritoneal Dialysis Nurse
**CPNP**   Certified Pediatric Nurse Practitioner
**CPON**   Certified Pediatric Oncology Nurse
**CPSN**   Certified Plastic Surgical Nurse
**CRNA**   Certified Registered Nurse Anesthetist
**CRNH**   Certified Registered Nurse Hospice
**CRNI**   Certified Registered Nurse Intravenous
**CRNO**   Certified Registered Nurse in Ophthalmology
**CRNP**   Certified Registered Nurse Practitioner
**CRRN**   Certified Rehabilitation Registered Nurse
**CSN**   Certified School Nurse
**CURN**   Certified Urology Registered Nurse

**BOX 2-1—cont'd**

**CWCN**   Certified Wound Care Nurse
**FPN**   Family Nurse Practitioner
**GNP**   Gerontological Nurse Practitioner
**NMCC**   National Managed Care Certification
**OGNP**   Obstetric/Gynecological Nurse Practitioner
**ONC**   Oncology Nurse Certified
**PNP**   Pediatric Nurse Practitioner
**RNC**   Registered Nurse Certified
**RN,CNA**   Registered Nurse, Certified in Nursing Administration
**RN,CNAA**   Registered Nurse, Certified in Nursing Administration, Advanced
**RN,CS**   Registered Nurse, Certified Specialist

Are dates in order, or are there gaps? Is any information missing (information that you would expect the person to have—based on other entries in the resumé)? Are the expected licenses and certifications listed? Do the educational entries and on-the-job training support skills mentioned elsewhere? Is equipment used in this position noted in the resumé? Are there obvious entries or claims that call for verification? Is the spelling correct? Are technical entries used in the correct context? Is it obvious that the candidate has been keeping up on the technical aspects of healthcare? Has the person performed in a similar role or functional area? If the position in question represents a promotion, does the person have the requisite experience, continuing education, and background to justify such a promotion? For instance, certain positions today require budget experience.

Although the resumé is a marketing document designed to make the candidate look good, the interview "detective" should gather a number of clues for interview questions.

The same approach applies to the application. Many companies do not allow the applicant to write "see resumé" on the application. There are several reasons, the most important of which is that the applicant does not sign the resumé.

The application is a signed document that usually states, close to the signature block, that the applicant affirms the information above to be true and gives the prospective employer the right to check the veracity of all statements. Erroneous statements made on the application can be sufficient reason for termination.

Note the candidate's time in his or her current position, reasons for leaving, and position title. Does the time look right? Is the reason for leaving a desire for advancement, or is the person a "job hopper?" Keep in mind that certain organizations require rapid movement, particularly when the individual is in a learning mode. This, of course, should be reflected in the "reason for leaving" column. Is there any hint that the person may have been asked to leave? Has the person been in similar positions long enough to acquire the experience required? Does the salary seem to be in range with the position? Do not let a previous high salary keep you from considering a candidate. On the other hand, if the position to be filled is a lesser one, would the person be happy with the challenge of the new position and, perhaps, with working for someone having less experience or education? Or would that person be gone in a short period, necessitating going through the hiring process again? Money is not always the deciding factor. However, you should try to uncover the candidate's motivation during the interview.

It is incumbent on the organization to establish the applicant's eligibility to work in the United States. All employees must complete an I-9 form to ascertain their legal work status. If the potential employee cannot provide proof of eligibility within 3 days of hiring, that person is not eligible to work. As in the resumé, you must check for the required licenses and certifications or verify that the applicant has applied for the necessary documentation.

Most applications ask for references. Who are the best references? From the potential employer's point of view, they are is those who will honestly speak of the person's ability to function in the type of position being filled. A current problem is that the specter of lawsuits hangs over the giving of references. Many large organizations prohibit their employees from giving references for departing employees. This situation makes the entire reference process fraught with uncertainty. Adding to the confusion is the fact that some companies hire outside agencies to do records and reference checks. (The stories of information given during reference checks would fill volumes of script material for "Saturday Night Live.") One approach you might try is to ask a provided reference for the name of another acquaintance of the person being checked. Then call that person and ask your reference-check questions.

The next thing to check for is *longevity.* Add up the number of years/months that the applicant has worked in each job. Has the person stayed only a few months? Combine that information with the reason given for leaving to determine what the chances are that the applicant will stay with your company. Be careful of job hoppers. These are employees who stay with a company just long enough to get their bonuses without repayment of benefits and then leave for another company with a bonus. Just because an employee has had several jobs within a short number of years does not always point to job hopping. Some positions require you to change positions to continue up the "ladder of success."

Next, consider the *number of years/months of experience in the necessary skills* of the vacant position. If an application shows a very similar type of skill, award the full time at that previous job. If the application indicates a somewhat similar type of skill, award half the time of the previous job. In that way everyone is credited with the same selective process.

Look at the applicant's *salary history.* Many managers see an applicant who has made, or is making, much more money than they could offer. Do not let that stop you from considering an applicant. If the application or resumé does not offer an insight as to why the applicant would consider a lesser-paying position, note that as one of your questions if you decide to interview that person.

## DOCUMENTATION FOR EVALUATING CLIENTS AND RECORD KEEPING

To stay organized, to ensure equity, and to document justification of your decision, it is important to keep accurate records. Selecting the wrong person for the job is extremely costly. Resolving hiring errors can frequently lead to lawsuits with their attendant negative publicity. Avoiding that situation is the preferred method. First, construct an evaluation sheet based on the tasks to be performed in the position. It is best to fill out the evaluation sheet during or immediately after the interview. Such documentation is important to back up your position on why a candidate was hired or not hired. Of all the onerous paperwork a manager needs to do, personnel documentation is the most unpopular.

### Sample Organizational Tips

#### *Labels*

Make labels to go on the back of each application with the following information:

| Last Name, First Name | Date of Application |
| Position Applied For | |
| | |
| Years/Months of Experience: | |
| Education: | Specialties: |

#### *Checklist*

Then create a checklist with the information taken from the label:

| Name | Experience | Education | Appearance | Attitude | Total |
|------|-----------|-----------|------------|----------|-------|
|      |           |           |            |          |       |
|      |           |           |            |          |       |

Information about appearance and attitude will be filled in after the interview.

## THE INTERVIEW

With as much as has been written about the interview, you would think that everyone has this step under control. They don't! First, what is the role of the manager during the interview? It is to determine which of the candidates fits best into the organization. "Fit" involves the mission, function, and personality of the existing organization. Question and test all candidates to determine which, if any, fits best into your organization. This is not something that can be done well quickly or without preparation.

The setting for the interview is very important. If it is to be conducted one-on-one in an office, behind the desk ("I'm king and you can't dethrone me!") is *not* where the manager should sit. Try using two equal chairs separated by an end table, with adequate lighting, coffee, tea, soft drinks, and *no* interruptions. The same preparations should be made even if the setting is a conference room with a team interview approach (very popular in some companies today).

Begin the interview with a description of the position and the institution. Make sure that the applicant is fully aware of the most important factors of the job—the duties and requirements and how they relate to the functioning of the unit. Remember, you are trying to sell the position to the applicant as much as the applicant is trying to sell his or her services to you. In preparation, jot down a few important reasons why the applicant should consider the position.

### Hints for a Productive Interview

- Select a quiet, private area if possible.
- Have all participants ready to start on time.
- Make sure everyone has a copy of the resumé, application, job description, job specification sheet, and the evaluation sheet.

- Keep the interview area neat and orderly.
- Arrange for no interruptions.
- Make sure the candidate is greeted and escorted to the interview location.
- Dress professionally. Keep in mind that one part of the interviewer's job is to persuade the candidate that he or she wants to work for your organization. You are "marketing" your institution.
- Be organized. Lack of organization is readily noticed and is often one of the first observations made by candidates.
- Try to make the candidate comfortable. Nervousness, even on the part of the interviewer(s), is to be expected.
- Keep to the time schedule, especially if you and/or the candidate have other interviews scheduled.
- Greet the candidate and introduce yourself. Then introduce the other interviewers.
- Shake hands with the interviewee, whether a man or a woman.
- Put the interviewee at ease by talking about something that puts you on common ground.

### Types of Questions to Be Included in the Interview

Develop clearly worded questions, and outline what you expect for answers. The interview should include informational questions, behavioral questions, and situational questions. Some examples of each follow.

#### *Informational questions*
- Why did you leave your last position?
- How did you find out about this job?
- Why did you apply for this position?
- In what way do you think you can contribute to the department?
- What would you say are the major qualities this job demands?
- What kind of work interests you most?
- What did you enjoy *most* about your last/present job?

- What did you enjoy *least* about your last/present job?
- What were the biggest pressures on your last job?
- If there were two things you could change in your last/present job, what would they be and how would you change them?
- If you could make one constructive suggestion to management, what would it be?
- What qualifications do you have that make you successful in this field?
- What aspects of your work do you consider most crucial?
- Of all the work you have done, where have you been most successful?
- What are the disadvantages of your chosen field?
- In your nurse's training, in what subject did you do best? Why?
- In your nurse's training, with what subject did you have the most trouble? Why?
- What prompted you to choose nursing as your major?
- Can you perform the duties required in this position? (Be *very* careful with this one. The *Americans With Disabilities Act* prohibits employers from discriminating against employees or applicants on the basis of disability. But let's face it—a health provider usually needs to be able to lift at least 40 pounds. Leave the expansion of this question to the applicant. If the applicant wants to tell you more than "yes" or "no," let the person do so. Do not ask further.)

### Behavioral questions

- Tell me what you did in a situation where you were faced with a deadline and additional demands were unexpectedly placed on you.
- Describe a time when you gained a patient's trust even though the patient was unresponsive at first.
- Tell me about some situations in which you went the "extra mile" to satisfy a patient.
- Tell me how you went about organizing your duties in your last job.

- What kind of people annoy you most?
- Have you ever been in a dispute with a supervisor? What was it about, and how was it resolved?
- Have you ever been in a dispute with a coworker? What was it about, and how was it resolved?

### Situational questions

- You have reported for work only to find that you are short-handed. You have a nursing assistant available for help. The lab is on the phone with the results of a test, a patient's buzzer has gone off, a physician is waiting to make his rounds with you, and you have an angry relative demanding to be updated on his grandmother immediately. What action would you take first, and why?
- You see a person at the hospital fall down a flight of stairs. What do you do?
- You have a patient whom you know personally, and you are aware he has AIDS. However, there is no indication in the medical records that the patient has AIDS. Do you alert anyone? If so, who?

Once you have selected the questions to be used, rehearse the interview. This technique can be very effective if you use your coworkers to provide input and feedback.

### Actual Interview Questions

There are several types of tough interview questions, and some are more appropriate to one employee classification level than to another. In many cases there is no "incorrect" answer, unless, of course, the candidate reveals something that completely rules out employment with your organization.

### Open-ended questions

In general, open-ended questions elicit more response than closed-ended questions (Fig. 2-1 and Box 2-2). However, good closed-ended questions can be used to help determine the "fit" across three areas: mission, function, and personality.

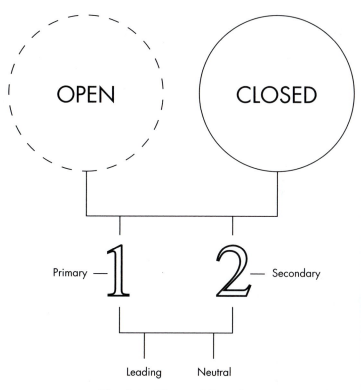

**Fig. 2-1**  Types of Questions.

- *Which do you prefer?*
  Tight deadlines/Loose timetables
  Written projects/Oral presentations
  Working alone/Working with others
- *Which best describes you?*
  Meticulous decision maker/Fast decision maker
  Conservative problem solver/Radical problem solver
  Generally a team member/Usually a leader
  Always busy/Generally busy
  Take initiative/Wait for orders
  Make suggestions/Wait to be asked

**BOX 2-2**

## PRIMARY AND SECONDARY QUESTIONS

| Primary | Secondary |
|---|---|
| **Definition** | **Definition** |
| These questions are used to introduce new topics for discussion. They can be open or closed in nature. | These questions are used to try to get more information or clarify a response. They are sometimes called "probing" or "follow-up" questions. |
| **Examples** | **Examples** |
| • How would you describe the ideal boss? | • Please continue |
| • What were your primary responsibilities in your last position? | • Which of these activities did you like best? |
| • What do you think are the most important characteristics of an effective clinical manager? | • Why do you think that is important? |
| **When to Use** | **When to Use** |
| • In the beginning of the interview to encourage openness | • After primary questions to encourage, clarify, probe, or follow-up |
| • To introduce a new line of questioning | |

The following are examples of open-ended questions and what the answers reveal.
- *How did you accomplish a tough task?* [Use one mentioned in the interview, or ask for an example.] *What steps did you take? Why did you choose them?* [Should reveal several skills, especially organizational, people, functional, etc.]
- *Where would you like to be 5 years from now?* [Indicate goal orientation, motivation.]
- *Suppose you had to work away from your area for an extended period of time. How would you feel about that?* [Shows adaptability.]

- *Describe one or two examples of your ability to work independently.* [Gives indication of independence, ability to work with little or no direct supervision, critical thinking, problem solving.]
- *Describe your greatest innovation at work.* [Shows creativity, problem-solving ability.]
- *What have you done to improve yourself professionally in the past 3 years?* [Indicates commitment to career growth, technical competency.]
- *Tell me about yourself.* (This is a universally hated question.) The interviewer thinks that this question will put the candidate at ease. It doesn't! In the worst case the candidate will reveal something that should not enter the interview (regarding spouse, children, religion, or age.) If you must use this question, modify it by adding more detail: *Tell me something about your professional background.*
- *Why are you leaving your current position?* Will the candidate reveal a professional or authority problem that would cloud or negate hiring this candidate?
- *What are your greatest strengths?* Are they realistic? Do they jibe with the resumé and application? Follow-up: *Why do you say that?* Are they the strengths you are seeking?
- *What is your greatest weakness?* The answer should indicate attitude, honesty. Does the candidate reveal a fatal hiring flaw by being brutally frank about a real or imagined shortcoming? Does the candidate indicate an effort, educational or otherwise, to overcome this weakness?
- *Describe a typical day on your last job.* This question really means: *Are you flexible? Can you shift gears and priorities quickly?* Two positive answers could come in response to this query: the candidate's reply may show a good grasp of the last position and indicate that changing priorities rapidly is expected and accomplished.
- *What did you like most about your last job?* Does the answer have any relationship to the new position? Did the candidate like anything about the previous position?
- *What did you like least about the last position?* Obviously, the answer should not be one of the critical elements of the new

position, although you would be surprised at how many times that is the case.

- *Why should I hire you?* The usual answer is "Because I'm qualified." The person should recap his or her skills and experience in line with the needs of the advertised position. In other words, the answer should say: "I fit your needs. I have the education, experience, skills, and talents you are looking for to fill this position."
- *Why do you want to work for us?* Has the candidate done any homework on the organization? Does the candidate care where she or he works? Is the answer some completely "off the wall," inappropriate response?
- *Where would your last manager/supervisor say you need improvement?* This question is a play on the greatest-weakness question. It often throws candidates, but it should not. In today's world of rapidly expanding technology, we can all use improvement. What percentage of the capabilities of today's software is used by most of us? Very little. Yet there are many software features that would make our tasks easier if we only knew they were there and how to use them.
- *Would you describe a situation in which your work was criticized?* How does the candidate handle positive criticism?
- *How would you feel about more education?* In healthcare today competency is an important issue.
- *How would you describe your personality?* Do you want a "loner" in a team situation? Do you want someone who gets flustered when a family member asks an unexpected question? Does "laid back" mean "I don't get flustered," or does it mean lazy, with little or no motivation?
- *What do you do when your manager/supervisor tells you to do something you do not agree with?* This question is another attitude check. It assumes that there is nothing illegal or immoral in the directive, only a difference of opinion about what to do in a given situation or how to do it. The candidate should indicate that, based on education or experience, he or she would offer an alternate solution or

approach. However, if the boss said, "This is the way we're going to do it," then the boss would have 100% support. (There is always time to question the boss in a positive, I-want-to-learn manner, later.)

- *What is the most difficult thing you have had to do in your present or previous job?* Again, this is a wide-open invitation to reveal a skill, knowledge, or personality shortcoming. Resist the trap of asking the question as: "Do you have any difficulty with . . . ?" This closed-ended question is too easy for the candidate and in most cases reveals nothing.

- *Give me an example of a task you had to do under pressure. How did you do it?* Here you are looking for an answer that indicates the candidate's organizational skills and functional abilities. An attitude problem might also surface.

### *Situational questions*

Because customer service to the patient, the patient's family, and the medical staff is so important, it is wise to have a few situational questions ready to ask. These should invite the candidate to problem-solve (think critically) and give you an indication of the person's logical thinking and ethics. Questions about a conflict with a co-worker and how it was handled or how a difficult patient was calmed or an irate family member was satisfied frequently elicit "telling" responses. These are responses telling you there is a problem. The candidate may reveal a negative attitude toward these situations, may show little concern for customer service, or may not think logically to solve problems. Even worse, the candidate may tell you, directly or indirectly, that customer service is not part of his or her job!

Other functional areas should be explored through situational or *Tell me about your experience with* . . . questions. In certain technical situations it is a good idea to have the person demonstrate equipment operation. A certain type of candidate will have "no problem" with any situation or equipment you mention. The liberal translation is that there is a problem, and you had better be on your toes!

Another common eye-opener is *Describe the ideal working situation for you.* Almost any good working environment trait(s) could be mentioned, such as up and down communications, supportive atmosphere, advancement possibilities, or continuing education opportunities. Beware if you get any answers that include "top pay, short hours," "nobody on my back," and similar flippant replies, which are probably indicative of a problem attitude.

*What manager did you like most?* and *What manager did you like least?* should elicit very professional no-name responses revolving around a good "managerial" working environment or lack of one. The answer to these questions may indicate a negative attitude toward authority, a lack of professionalism, an inability to get along with certain people (possibly based on sex, race, or religion).

### Questions That *Cannot* Be Asked

The general rule is to stick to topics directly related to the job. Stay away from questions about the candidate's marital status or children (e.g., with whom the children live, or what their ages are). Questions regarding nationality, race, or religious affiliation, even of a school attended, are not pertinent. As the following examples show, how you phrase a question can make all the difference in the world.

| | |
|---|---|
| CORRECT: | Do you have 20/20 corrected vision? |
| INCORRECT: | What is your corrected vision? |
| CORRECT: | How well can you handle stress? |
| INCORRECT: | Does stress ever affect your ability to be productive? |
| CORRECT: | How many days were you absent from work last year? |
| INCORRECT: | How many days were you sick last year? |

| CORRECT: | Are you currently using illegal drugs? |
| INCORRECT: | What medications are you currently taking? |
| CORRECT: | Do you drink alcohol? |
| INCORRECT: | How much alcohol do you drink per week? |

Do not ask open-ended questions about memberships in clubs and other organizations, for example, "To which clubs do you belong?" It should be noted that large companies often seek favor in the community by having employees who are active in community and community-supportive organizations. Since nurse managers could find themselves in health maintenance organizations (HMOs), large insurance companies, public and private prison systems, and similar organizations, it is a good area to check with human resources for the latest legal guidance in this area. Otherwise, mention the names and types of neutral community organizations that the company promotes and see if the candidate responds that he or she is currently a member or is interested in joining such an organization.

Illegal questions are those associated with age, religion, nationality, and sexual orientation. *Never* ask the following questions:

- How old are you?
- Do you have any children?
- Do you go to church?
- What nationality are you?

**Focus on Objectives**

The following tips are designed to help you achieve the results you want from the interview. Most important, keep your objectives in mind throughout the process.

1. Consider who will fit best into your organization, according to its mission, function, and personality.
2. Provide enough information about the organization so that the candidate can make an informed decision.

3. Keep the other interviewer role—salesperson for the organization—foremost in your mind.

4. Once you determine that the candidate does fit into your organization, sell the person on taking the job.

Before you begin interviewing, prepare a series of questions that probe the specific tasks and requirements for the position. Be ready for spontaneous follow-up questions. This style is often referred to as the semistructured interview.

Allow sufficient time for the interview. You will develop a better feel for the time required for you or your team to conduct a thorough interview after going through at least two interviews for the various types of positions in your unit. In general, allow 30 minutes for unskilled or semiskilled positions. For managerial, professional (exempt level, not necessarily a manager), and highly skilled technical positions, allow 1 hour. These guidelines do not mean that the time allotted must be used, as long as all the candidates are asked enough of the standard questions to form a basis for comparison. Do *not* let interviews drag, and do not let one team member dominate the questioning. Throughout the interview, jot down key words and phrases used by the candidate. Note whether the applicant makes eye contact, keeping in mind that it is perfectly normal for people to look away while formulating their response and then to resume eye contact. Observers and tape recorders are not permitted. Do not criticize or become argumentative with the candidate. Their response could be to try to tell you what they think you want to hear, negating the entire interview.

Immediately after the interview, review all pertinent data regarding the candidate: application, resumé, test scores, interviewers' comments, references, evaluation sheets, and job specification sheets.

Research on interviews has shown the following:

1. Interviewers form an opinion of the candidate within the first few seconds of the interview.

2. Interviewers who are experiencing pressure to hire have a tendency to rate candidates higher than those who are not feeling such pressure.

3. The more the interviewer knows about the position being filled, the better "fit" the interviewer is inclined to make.

4. When evaluating candidates, interviewers tend to contrast candidates with previous ones; therefore an applicant with average qualifications will be rated lower if he or she is immediately preceded by a candidate having above-average qualifications.

5. Interviewers develop a stereotype of the "ideal" candidate against which all candidates are evaluated. (Overcome this tendency by focusing on the documentation previously mentioned, especially a good job description.)

6. Because several candidates "look good on paper," the selection interview can become a search for negative, rather than positive, information, with the negative carrying more weight.

## CANDIDATE EVALUATION

Try to make your evaluation immediately after the interview. If you wait, it is more likely that your evaluation will be based on impressions rather than fact. Evaluate the candidate(s) based on the checklists, not "off the cuff." There is no perfect candidate. It is highly unlikely that any one candidate will have all the skills, education, experience mix, and interpersonal skills you have specified. Therefore it is very important that you have followed your checklists and made relevant comments. If the interview was conducted using the team concept (whether the interviews were conducted separately or as a group), collect oral and written comments from the "team" as soon as possible.

### Narrowing the Selection

Using a combination of the requirements advertised for the position and the individual information you gathered, select at least the top ten applicants. From these top ten, rate the

## Management Spotlight

### *MAKE SURE YOU MAKE A DIFFERENCE*

- People who make the team are supposed to make a difference.
- Contribute in such a way that one clearly adds value.

From Pritchett, P. (1997). *The team member handbook for teamwork.*
Dallas: Pritchett & Associates.

top five from that group. Never interview too many applicants. After more than five continuous interviews, it is easy to forget who was whom. Make a note about why each selection was made. This information can be very beneficial if you become involved in a hiring dispute. From the top five candidates, you are now ready to check their references.

### Checking References

Check past employment references. Write down a few questions that you want to be sure to ask of each reference. The following are sample questions:

- With whom am I speaking, and what is your title?
- What was your relationship to the applicant?
- How long did the applicant work for you? (This question should be answered on the application or resumé, but it is a good idea to verify that the length of service is approximately the same).
- Is this applicant eligible for rehire? (This is one of the most important questions you can ask. Many companies are hesitant to give you any information about a former employee, but the majority will at least answer this question.)
- Did the applicant hold any other positions with the company?
- How would you describe his or her work ethic?

- What reservations should I have about hiring him or her?
- What were the reasons the applicant left your company?

## CANDIDATE FOLLOW-UP

- Do not delay. The longer the period between the interview and your follow-up, the more likely you are to lose the candidate.
- Keep in close contact with your organization's recruiters and human resources personnel.
- Provide the recruiters with your evaluation of each candidate as quickly as possible. Let your manager know of particularly impressive candidates in case he or she wants to interview them.
- Do not leave the candidate "hanging." Make sure that someone on the recruiting team has been in touch if that was promised.
- If you want to interview the candidate again, arrange for the follow-up interview as quickly as possible.
- If the decision is to not offer a position, make sure that the candidate is notified quickly and in a professional manner.
- The details of any offer should be worked out with the manager, human resources, and the recruiting team as soon as possible.
- Do not delay in notifying the candidate of the offer. Good performers often have other options and may be off the job market quickly.
- Keep in mind that you have just spent a good deal of effort in securing this employee. Now, how do you keep this person motivated and happy?

## SALARY

Normally, the total compensation package is administered by human resources. Total compensation includes medical, eye, dental, and disability insurance and similar benefits. Also included are vacation, sick, and personal days and paid holidays. Benefit packages vary from institution to institution and by employee level. Generally, the organization has a policy on the scale for all positions and on the increases that can be offered based on education, experience, shift differential, weekend hours, and other incentive programs. These are fairly rigid to avoid charges of favoritism; they also could be set forth in union contracts. Follow the guidelines provided by human resources.

If it should become obvious that you are not attracting high-quality candidates because the salary offering is below that of the competition (and you can prove that), go to human resources with a counterproposal on the compensation package. Senior-level employees often want something other than salary increases. More vacation, increased benefit options (especially in savings and retirement plans), stock options, and similar "perks" are often more popular with senior-level workers, especially when tax breaks are part of the equation.

## MAKING THE OFFER

When you are ready to make the offer, it is best to have an "offer script" written (Box 2-3). You need to keep your offer as basic as possible in case of a dispute. If questions are asked about the offer that are not on the offer script, it is recommended that you tell the person you will get back with them on the specifics of the unanswered question. Keep the completed script on file for possible reference.

First, date the script, and list the name and phone number of the person to whom the offer will be made. Next, list the position title and number (for internal use only), followed by the salary and major benefits.

Ask if the person will accept the offer. If the answer is "yes," repeat the position title and salary and set the start date. Make sure that the candidate knows about orientation, if applicable, and the pay and hours for the orientation (if different from the normal salary and working hours). Do not begin your relationship with this individual with a major unpleasant surprise!

**BOX 2-3**

## SAMPLE OFFER SCRIPT

May I speak to _____. Hi, this is _____, and I'd like to make you an offer for the _____ position at _____ for a salary of _____.
This offer is contingent on your being licensed for the state of _____ and completing our employee health program.

Would you like for me to go over the benefits of the position?

We offer _____ days vacation after the _____, and sick leave is accumulated at _____ per pay period. We offer medical and dental insurance at the rate of _____ for individual coverage and _____ for family coverage. We have a 401(k) plan, a tuition reimbursement, and in-house training for ACLS.

Would you be interested in accepting our offer? Yes/No If no, ask why. If it's salary, ask how much they are looking for. (If it's within that minimum/maximum range, you can negotiate from here; if not, tell them you will get back with them after you see if their salary desires can be met.)

If they accept, set the start date. If they are currently employed, they may need to give a 2-week notice. If they need to relocate, it could be up to a month or more.

Explain the processing the new employee will need to do, and set dates to start this processing. Ask if they have any questions. Give them your name and phone number in case they need to contact you again before their first day with the company.

Human Resource Principles

Give your name and work number to the new employee. Ask if the person has any questions, and then reiterate the start date and time: "I look forward to seeing you Monday, at 8 AM, in the conference room. Parking is available in the west visitors parking lot until you receive a parking sticker during orientation." These details can mean a lot to the new employee in regard to starting off on the right foot and feeling welcome.

For certain positions (usually exempt level), a formal *offer letter* is appropriate and should be extended to the candidate.

Human resources has the format. Frequently this letter is controlled by human resources because of its content and legal considerations. The letter reiterates the position title, salary, and location. Any contingencies are also noted. Requirements that must be completed, such as licenses or a health examination, are listed. Relocation and reimbursement terms are detailed in case the employee does not meet the minimum length of stay specified. The offer letter does *not* constitute an employment contract, and you should avoid any mention of a contract. The letter needs to be signed by the employee and filed in the employment jacket. Even though the individual may have verbally indicated an intention to accept your offer, it is not unusual to have an offer letter declined.

If the answer to your verbal offer is "no", that is the time to ask pertinent questions. Use a friendly approach to elicit the information you need: "I realize you're a busy person. I do need your assistance in solving my staffing problem. What specifically is the reason [or reasons] for not accepting the position? Is the major problem salary?" Naturally, open-ended questions are preferred; however, there are times when, with the "right" individuals, a closed-ended query will start a flow of information.

## EMPLOYMENT LAWS

1. *Americans With Disabilities Act* prohibits employers from discriminating against an employee because of a permanent disability. The law requires an employer to make reasonable accommodation to the known physical or mental limitations of an otherwise qualified applicant or employee, unless it can be shown that the accommodation would cause an undue hardship on the employer's operations.

2. *Title VII of the Civil Rights Act of 1964* is the basic federal law prohibiting discrimination in employment. It has been amended several times since it was first enacted. This law prohibits discrimination based on race, color, national origin, religion, sex, and pregnancy.

3. *Age Discrimination in Employment Act* bars discrimination in employment against persons age 40 and over.

4. *Family Medical Leave Act* requires employers of 50 or more workers to provide up to 12 weeks per year for an employee to care for a newborn or newly adopted child; to care for a seriously ill spouse, parent, or child; or because of the employee's own illness. Employers are prohibited from discriminating against employees who exercise their leave rights.

5. *Equal Pay Act* requires an employer to pay men and women at the same rate for equal work.

6. *Vietnam Era Veterans' Readjustment Assistance Act* and prior laws protect the jobs of reservists and employees called to active duty in the armed forces.

7. *Immigration Reform and Control Act* requires employers to verify employment authorization of newly hired employees. It requires two types of documentation, right to work and identity.

Nearly all states and many counties and municipalities have enacted their own fair employment practices laws. These laws often extend the coverage of the basic federal statute.

## COUNSELING

If you ever find it necessary to counsel an employee, remember the three rules: document, document, and document. From the very beginning it is necessary to document your actions. Have you spoken directly to the employee? Have you spelled out for the person what is required by the position description and where the individual is falling short? Have you set a time limit for improvement and explained the type and degree of improvement expected? Is this information documented? Was the follow-up actually conducted? Did the person ask for reasonable assistance, and was it provided? Once it became obvious that the situation was not getting any better, was human resources notified? Did you ascertain whether or not the employee knew of assistance available through employee assistance program (EAP)?

Once human resources is involved, the manager is generally following very specific guidelines and documenting procedures. These must be completed as set forth in the personnel manual. Failure to do so will potentially jeopardize any actions taken against the employee. It may also leave the manager open for criticism. As with all personnel actions, positive professional steps must be taken the entire way. If you start with the correct approach, maintain contact with human resources, and follow the established procedures, you will have much less difficulty in dealing with the ever-changing field of employee relations.

## BIBLIOGRAPHY

Institute for International Research. (1996). *Understanding the fundamentals of personnel law.* Walnut Creek, CA: Council on Education in Management.

Levesque, J. D. (1991). *The complete hiring manual.* Englewood Cliffs, NJ: Prentice-Hall.

Peabody & Brown. (1994). Labor, employment and benefits. In *Peabody & Brown Report* (Winter), Internet.

Peters, T., & Austin, N. (1991). *A passion for excellence.* New York: Random House.

Swansburg, R. (1990). *Management and leadership for nurse managers.* Boston: Jones & Bartlett.

Wendover, R. (1995). *Smart hiring.* Naperville, IL: Sourcebooks.

# Chapter 3

# Management Principles

## Problem Solving and Employee Performance Appraisals

*H*alf of our mistakes in life arise from feeling where we
ought to think and thinking where we ought to feel.

*John C. Collins*

With the increasing complexity and turbulence of healthcare
changes, individuals in leadership roles must learn to analyze
situations quickly and make sound decisions. Problem-solving
models and quality improvement tools are available to assist
an individual in organizing data. It is important to identify the
underlying dynamics or root causes of a problem to reap long-
term benefits from the improvement initiative. If the underlying dynamics are not addressed, it is possible that only a
symptom of the problem will be corrected.

Sometimes it is assumed that innate abilities, educational
levels, past experiences, and intuition form the basis for successful decisions. It can be difficult to choose among known
alternatives; yet how much more difficult it is to choose
among unknown alternatives. The process of decision making
contains many sequenced steps. Making a choice is just one
element. Another dimension to decision making is putting
the choice into action.

Constructing simple models or applying scientific methods
to the field of quality can reduce any problem to its significant
components. Once a problem is reduced within a model, it
usually can be more easily visualized and subsequently

---

**Management Spotlight**

*INSTEAD OF CHANGING TEAMS, HELP CHANGE THE TEAM THAT YOU ARE ALREADY IN. . . . START WITH YOURSELF!*

If you want to play on a championship team, or work with a high performance unit, you cannot afford to be an ordinary performer.

From Pritchett, P. (1997). *The team member handbook for teamwork.* Dallas: Pritchett & Associates.  •

---

understood. Although there are many decision-making models in the literature, the following depict user-friendly and frequently used models.

## PROBLEM-SOLVING MODELS
### Steps in the Process

Most models identify five basic steps in the problem-solving process. *First,* the problem must be identified. Collecting factual information and perceptions is essential. Swansburg (1990) suggests three approaches to prioritizing problems:
- Deal with problems in the order in which they appear.
- Solve the easiest problems first.
- Solve crisis problems before all others.

The *second* step is gathering and analyzing information related to the solution. This step involves defining specifications. One should know what current policies, procedures, and standard practice require. The *third* step is evaluating all alternatives. It is wise to have a multidisciplined group to participate in creating all possible alternatives. For each alternative, list both the positive and negative consequences. Disagreement may stimulate creativity to produce better solutions. The *fourth* step is to act on or implement the selected alternative. This includes sequencing of plans and communication for implementation. The *fifth* step is to monitor the implementation outcome and evaluate effectiveness. Progress needs to be monitored on an ongoing basis.

## The Descriptive Model

This model allows for the fact that many decisions are made with incomplete information because of time, money, or people limitations and recognizes that people do not always make good choices. Sound familiar? Steps in the descriptive model include the following (Swansburg, 1990):

1. Establish an acceptable goal.
2. Define the subjective perceptions of the problem.
3. Identify acceptable alternatives.
4. Evaluate each alternative.
5. Select an alternative.
6. Implement the decision.
7. Do follow-up.

## The PDCA Model

Healthcare organizations frequently define one scientific method in terms of the PDCA cycle (Schroeder, 1994). PDCA stands for *P*lan/*D*o/*C*heck/*A*ct:

### *Plan*
- Identify one's targeted customer groups.
- Identify the problem/process, and define the significant needs and characteristics that are important to the customer groups in relationship to the identified problem.
- Develop the product or service based on solutions that can meet the majority of these needs.

### *Do*
- Do the improvement.
- Identify costs, people, and materials.
- Educate management and staff.

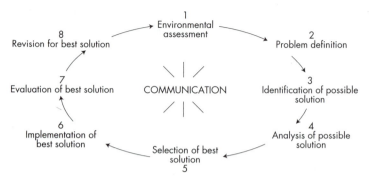

**Fig. 3-1** Basic Problem-Solving Model.

(From Strasen, L. [1987]. *Key business skills for nurse managers.* Philadelphia: Lippencott.)

### Check

- Check and study results through continuous analytical measurement.
- Contrast results to customer expectations and evaluations.

### Act

- Hold the gain.
- Continue to improve the process, system, or service.

Another basic problem-solving model is described by Strasen (1987), and is also depicted as a cycle (Fig. 3-1).

The acronyms, approaches, and models used all have similar steps and objectives. Table 3-1 compares the PDCA cycle with the problem-solving methods of the nursing process and a 10-step process used in many disciplines for monitoring quality.

Before acting on or implementing the selected alternative in the decision, it is important to ask the following seven questions to increase the chance of success (Swansburg, 1990):

1. Does the quality of the decision really make a difference?
2. Do I have all the information I need to make the decision alone?
3. Do I know what I am missing? Do I know where to find the information? Will I know what to do with the information I am given?

**Table 3-1**   Process Comparisons

| PDCA Cycle | 10-Step Process | Nursing Process |
|---|---|---|
| Plan | 1. Responsibility | Assess |
| | 2. Scope of care | Diagnose |
| | 3. Important aspects of care | Plan |
| | 4. Indicators | |
| | 5. Thresholds | |
| Do | 6. Collect data | Intervene |
| Check | 7. Evaluate | Evaluate |
| Act | 8. Take action | |
| | 9. Reassess | |
| | 10. Communicate findings | |

From Schroeder, P. (1994). *Improving quality and performance: Concepts, programs, and techniques.* St Louis: Mosby.

4. Do I need anybody's commitment to make sure this succeeds?
5. Can I gain commitments without offering participation in the decision?
6. Do those involved in the decision share the organization's goals?
7. Is there likely to be conflict about the available alternatives? If so, can I rank the pain factor associated with the implementation of each alternative?

## DECISION MAKING
### Pitfalls of Decision Making

Individual managers, as well as cultures, are still *resistant to change,* which involves taking risks and exploring new ideas. They may lack trust in others who will test new areas. If a manager chooses to control decision making and omits those affected by the decision from the process, the less likely others will be to commit to implementing the decision.

*Inadequate fact finding* will result in many unanticipated problems, which probably could have been avoided or solved.

During the outcomes monitoring phase, it will become evident that the decision may not have been the best solution, given other alternatives.

*Time constraints* present a huge challenge. Pressures of time, resources, and priorities render the decision-making process very complex. The risk assumed is greater when time is insufficient to produce adequate fact-finding information.

*Poor communication* yields many problems with all aspects of problem solving. The greater the communication, the higher will be the degree of certainty of expected results.

*Failing to systematically follow the steps* of the decision-making process/model can also produce unanticipated results.

### Improving Decision Making

Besides the basic concepts already identified, Swansburg (1990) mentions other issues related to optimal decision making. These include educating people to know how to make decisions and securing administration support. For decision making at the lowest possible level, it is necessary to (1) establish decision-making checkpoints with appropriate time limits, (2) keep informed of progress by ensuring access to first-hand information, and (3) use statistical analysis to determine the significance of outcomes.

In decision making, an effective manager is one who:

- Stays informed about decisions made at different levels in the organization.
- Delegates all responsibilities possible.
- Deals with only those decisions requiring his or her level of expertise (when possible).
- Supports the implementation of decisions and, more importantly, credits the decision maker.

Swansburg further asserts that managers who make all the decisions themselves convey a lack of trust in the ability or loyalty of their subordinates. Selective delegation of decision making gains the support of the staff and raises their self-esteem. A successful manager is a motivator who is skilled and knowledgeable in both decision making and problem solving and thus serves as a role model for others.

### The Role of Intuition in Decision Making

Intuitive reasoning abilities do indeed have a place in executive decision making. Intuition is simply the power to perceive the possibilities inherent in a situation accurately. According to the Myers-Briggs Type Indicator surveys, an individual who thinks intuitively has a sense of vision, generating new ideas and ingenious solutions to old problems. According to research stemming from follow-up of 200 executives, seven conditions (Swansburg, 1990) were identified in which intuitive ability seems to function best:

1. When a high level of uncertainty exists
2. When few previous precedents exists
3. When variables are less scientifically predictable
4. When facts are limited
5. When facts do not clearly point the direction to go
6. When analytical data are of little use
7. When several plausible alternative solutions exist from which to choose, with good arguments for each

### METHODS FOR ANALYZING ALTERNATIVES IN PROBLEM SOLVING
#### Qualitative and Quantitative Analysis

- *Qualitative analysis.* This approach is somewhat subjective because the manager's past experiences, judgment, and expertise are used for problem solving and decision making.
- *Quantitative analysis.* This method is more objective because various alternatives identified can be converted into numerical terms. By quantifying data, one can more easily prioritize the alternatives, as well as identify the strengths and weaknesses of each alternative.

For optimal decision making, a combination of both qualitative and quantitative methods is frequently used.

Management Principles

## Benchmarking

Benchmarking is the search for best practices, which leads to value-driven outcomes. In a managed care environment, *value driven* means striving for high-quality outcomes balanced with cost-effectiveness and prudent stewardship of resources for both the service provider and the consumer.

In healthcare, benchmarking is frequently done outside the healthcare industry. One example is customer service. Customer service Walt Disney style, for example, is a popular philosophy that healthcare organizations are readily emulating by consulting the Disney management staff for their educational needs.

Benchmarking offers the following benefits:

- Increased ability to meet end-user customer requirements and expectations
- Establishment of goals based on empirical knowledge and best-practice industry standards
- Determination of standardized measures of quality and productivity
- Better positioning for a managed care environment

The four types of benchmarking (Katz & Green, 1997) are the following:

1. *Internal:* Comparison of internal processes, such as those between service areas or comparisons before and after implementation of the performance improvement initiative
2. *Competitive:* Competitor-to-competitor comparisons for a specific process
3. *Functional:* Comparison of processes or indicators to similar indicators within the same industry; uses best-practice standards
4. *Generic:* Comparison of indicators and processes regardless of industry

Examples of frequently benchmarked indicators are costs per unit of service, patient satisfaction scores, staffing ratios,

## Management Spotlight

*EFFECTIVE TEAMS TURN DIVERSITY TO THE TEAM'S ADVANTAGE*

- Don't sideline someone that is different.
- Do your part to help others identify and benefit from its full set of people, resource, and talents.

From Pritchett, P. (1997). *The team member handbook for teamwork.* Dallas: Pritchett & Associates.

hours per unit of service, hospital readmission rates, delayed patient discharges, and patient interventions.

### Analytical Tools for Organizing, Planning, and Decision Making

#### GANTT charts (Fig. 3-2)

- Useful for planning, implementing, and managing special projects and programs
- Tasks or steps to be accomplished are identified on a vertical axis; time frames are plotted on a horizontal axis
- Can be simple or extremely detailed
- Easily constructed to visualize the entire project
- Foster formal goal setting with target deadlines to attain goals

#### PERT charts

The PERT, or Program Evaluation and Review Technique, was developed specifically to keep track of the thousands of individual tasks in a special Navy project in the 1950s. The PERT chart is a network model or logistic method for displaying the relationships between activities and events to attain a specific program or project goal (Fig. 3-3).

Management Principles

| | Jul | Aug | Sep | Oct | Nov | Dec | Jan | Feb | Mar | Apr | May |
|---|---|---|---|---|---|---|---|---|---|---|---|
| 1. 3S consolidated with 3C <br> 4N consolidated with 4S | X <br> X | | | | | | | | | | |
| 2. Taskforce meetings (redesign created) | | X | X | X | | | | | | | |
| 3. Communications with staff; MDs (Unit meetings, Town Hall meetings, Medical Dept & multidisciplinary support meetings) | | X | X | X | X | | | | | | |
| 4. Nurse Manager Consolidation | | | | X | | | | | | | |
| 5. NRC Approval Facilities Planning Approval | | | | X | | | | | | | |
| 6. Punch out list distributed to ancillary support managers (cost analysis) | | | | X | X | | | | | | |
| 7. Employees on 2W, 3C, 3S, & 4N reapplied for positions | | | | X | X | | | | | | |
| 8. Employees offered positions (Beginning 11/21) | | | | | X | | | | | | |
| 9. Intense cleaning on 3S; painting patient rooms | | | | | X | | | | | | |
| 10. Moving 4S to 3S 11/22; (closing 4th floor) ~ decreased volume ~ holiday suggested by physicians ~ will give staff a chance to get "settled" prior to actual consolidation of staff/patient populations | | | | | X | | | | | | |
| 11. Continuing education/ competencies (See second page for specifics) | | | | X | X | X | X | | | | |
| 12. Staff/patient population consolidation, 12/10 | | | | | | X | | | | | |
| 13. Office/Storeroom to be converted to pt rooms (3S) Lounge/tx room converted to two patient rooms (3C) | | | | | | | X | X | | | |
| 14. Ambulatory Infusion Center (Old Peds Area) Projected Opening | | | | | | | | X | | | |
| 15. Annual competency fair | | | | | | | | | X | | |
| 16. MD/PT satisfaction tool specifically for Med/surg units | | | | | | | | | | X | X |

**Fig. 3-2**   Sample GANTT Chart:
Medical/Surgical Consolidation Plan

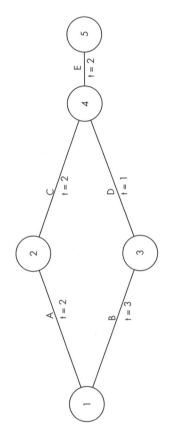

Opening of Ambulatory Infusion Center

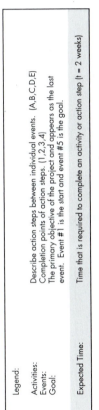

Legend:

| | |
|---|---|
| 1 | Develop orientation program |
| 2 | Interview qualified applicants |
| 3 | Select and schedule qualified applicants |
| 4 | Orient new employees |
| 5 | Open new patient care service area |

Activities: Describe action steps between individual events. (A,B,C,D,E)
Events: Completion points of action steps. (1,2,3,4)
Goal: The primary objective of the project and appears as the last event. Event #1 is the start and event #5 is the goal.

Expected Time: Time that is required to complete an activity or action step (t = 2 weeks)

**Fig. 3-3** Sample PERT Chart.

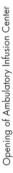

Management Principles

The PERT chart, which is more complex than a GANTT chart, is used primarily to:

- Identify deadlines for projects
- Identify individual events and activities required to meet a goal
- Establish realistic time lines

### Pareto principle and charts

The Pareto principle represents problem-solving efficiency. The emphasis is placed on capturing the few activities that count for most of the total effect or have the greatest impact. This principle correlates with the 80/20 rule: 80% of problems usually stem from only 20% of the causes or issues. An example of the Pareto principle: In the twenty steps in the preoperative admission process, only four of the steps account for 80% of the physician complaints.

A Pareto chart is a tool for prioritizing problems, the causes of a problem, or the categories of events and issues (Fig. 3-4). It can help a team focus on those issues that will have the greatest impact if they are solved.

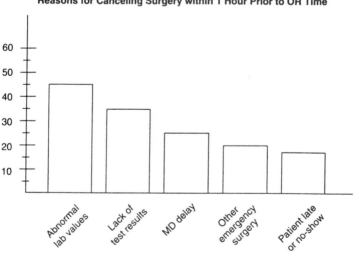

**Fig. 3-4**   Sample Pareto Chart.

(From Schroeder, P. [1994]. *Improving quality and performance.* St. Louis, MO: Mosby.)

### *Cause-and-effect diagrams (fishbone diagram)*

The fishbone diagram is an analytical tool used by teams to identify, explore, and graphically display the detailed possible causes related to a problem or condition and to discover its root causes (Fig. 3-5). This approach:

- Enables one to focus on the content of the problem, not its history, or the personal interests of team members
- Creates a "snapshot" of the collective knowledge and team consensus of a problem and subsequent support for the yielded solutions
- Focuses on causes and cures of problems/issues, not symptoms

### *Histograms*

A histogram is a visual picture used to summarize data from a process collected over time. It graphically presents its frequency distribution in bar form (Fig. 3-6).

This tool:

- Displays large amounts of data that are difficult to interpret in tabular form
- Illustrates the relative frequency, variations, and underlying distributions of the data
- Provides useful information for predicting future performance of the process

### *Force-field analysis*

Force-field analysis is used to analyze a situation or assist with a change in process (Fig. 3-7). It identifies factors in place that either support or work against the solution of an issue or problem. The positions can then be reinforced or the negatives can be eliminated or minimized. In addition, force-field analysis encourages honest reflection on the real underlying dynamics of a problem and its solution.

### *Flow charts*

Flow charts offer a wide range of applications. They can be used to create a picture of a process of care or service (Figs. 3-8 and 3-9). Flow charts:

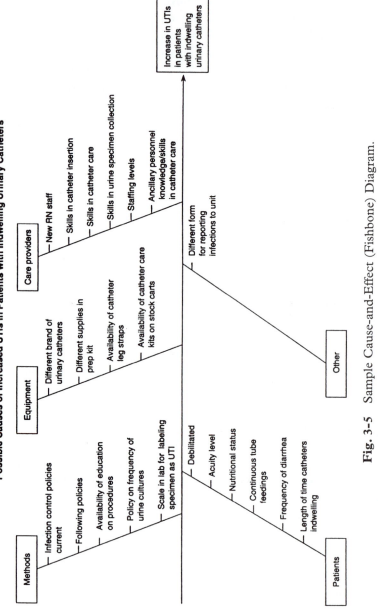

**Fig. 3-5**   Sample Cause-and-Effect (Fishbone) Diagram.
(From Schroeder, P. [1994]. *Improving quality and performance.* St. Louis, MO: Mosby.)

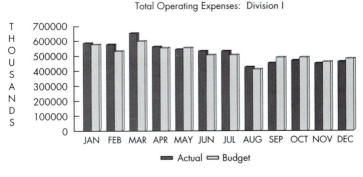

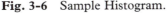

**Fig. 3-6**   Sample Histogram.

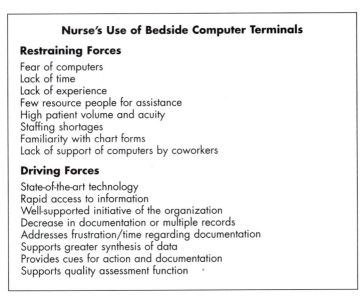

**Fig. 3-7**   Sample Force Field Analysis.

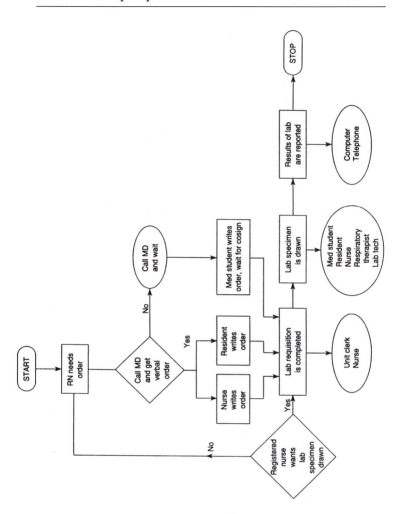

**Fig. 3-8** Sample Detailed Flow Chart.

(From Schroeder, P. [1994]. *Improving quality and performance*. St. Louis, MO: Mosby.)

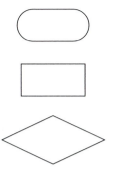

Oval is used to show the information or action (input) to start the process or to show the results at the end (output) of the process.

A box or rectangle is a step in the process.

A diamond illustrates a decision point.

**Fig. 3-9**   Symbols Used in Flow Charts.

- Identify unexpected complexity, problem areas, redundancy, and opportunities for standardization
- Compare and contrast the actual process with the benchmarked "best practice" process
- Serve as educational tools for understanding the complete process

### Tree diagrams
Tree diagrams are used to break down a goal or problem into manageable tasks (Fig. 3-10). These tools:
- Assist one to focus from a broad issue to specific components
- Serve as a guide for further analysis, planning, and implementation of the performance improvement initiative

### Nominal Group Technique
Nominal Group Technique (NGT) is not classified as an analytical tool. However, it is an activity commonly used to facilitate team decision making (Fig. 3-11). NGT is an approach that can bring a team to consensus quickly on the relative importance of issues, problems, or solutions by using individual priority rankings to develop a team priority matrix.

The NGT approach helps to:
- Build commitment to the team's choice through equal participation in the process.
- Force major causes of disagreement to be discussed.

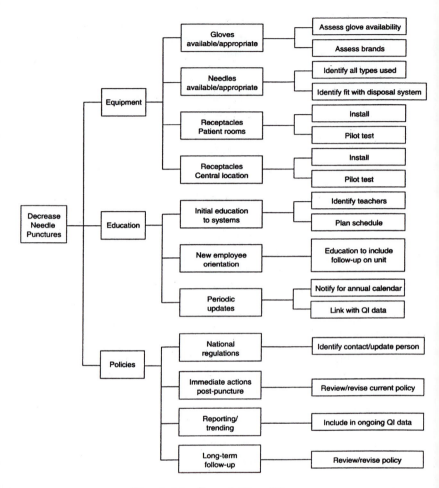

**Fig. 3-10**   Sample Tree Diagram.

(From Schroeder, P. [1994]. *Improving quality and performance*. St. Louis, MO: Mosby.)

### *Solution analysis*

Fig. 3-12 is an example of a solution analysis grid that is frequently used by all levels of management. Solution analysis grids are tools that assist a manager to detail objective, cost, feasibility, and time frames. As alternative solutions are visualized, the best acceptable solution is then selected.

**Example:** Why does the service area have a high percentage of noncompliance in patient teaching?
A. Lack of training
B. No documentation process
C. Unclear standards and expectations
D. High turnover in staff

| Criteria | Nurse 1 | Nurse 2 | Nurse 3 | Total |
|----------|---------|---------|---------|-------|
| A. | 4 | 5 | 1 | 10 |
| B. | 5 | 4 | 4 | 13 |
| C. | 3 | 3 | 2 | 8 |
| D. | 1 | 3 | 2 | 6 |

**Criteria B:** *No documentation process* would be the highest priority in this scenario.

**Fig. 3-11**    Sample Nominal Group Technique.

## CONSIDERATIONS IN PROBLEM SOLVING

It stands to reason that any problem resolution needs to be compatible with the philosophy and mission of the organization (*Action Tips* box). To determine the optimum alternatives, the following considerations should be identified:
- Timing
- Budget
- History and external factors
- Organizational vision, mission, and strategic objectives
- Interdepartmental impact
- Healthcare trends

## THE PERFORMANCE APPRAISAL PROCESS
### Manager's Preparation for the Performance Appraisal Interview*

As for any meeting, planning is the key to success. The performance appraisal interview has two components: process and content. The process consists of the format and the

---

*Modified from Umiker, W. (1995). Management skills for the new health care supervisor. In H. Rowland & B. Rowland, Nursing administration manual. Rockville, MD: Aspen Publishers.

**PROCEDURE**

1. *Contribution to Objective.* In this column, rank the alternative's contribution to the problem-solving objective using the qualifiers *high, medium,* and *low.*
2. *Cost in Dollars.* In this column, estimate the cost for preparation and implementation of the alternative. Use the symbols of three dollar marks ($$$), two dollar marks ($$), or one dollar mark ($) to indicate relative estimated dollar amounts.
3. *Time Frame.* In this column, estimate the amount of time it will take to prepare and implement a program that might

result from the alternative. Use the qualifiers *long-range, short-range,* and *immediate.*
4. *Feasibility.* In this column, enter *yes* or *no.* An affirmative or negative answer should be based on the decision-making constraints of the organization. Use a process of elimination to delete all alternatives that are deemed *not feasible.* Delete those alternatives that have a low contribution to the objective. Retain those alternatives that have a high or moderate contribution to the objective.

**GRID**

Problem-Solving Objective: _____

Problem Statement: _____

| Alternative Solutions | Contribution to Objective | Cost in Dollars | Time Frame | Feasibility |
|---|---|---|---|---|
| | | | | |
| | | | | |
| | | | | |
| | | | | |
| | | | | |
| | | | | |
| **Best Acceptable Solution:** | | | | |

**Fig. 3-12**    Solution Analysis Grid.

(From Umiker, W. [1995]. Management skills for the new health care supervisor. In H. Rowland & B. Rowland: *Nursing Administration manual.* Rockville, MD: Aspen Publishers.)

# Action Tips

## PROCEDURE FOR SOLVING PROBLEMS
## (SEVEN STEPS FOR PROBLEM RESOLUTION)

The following is a step-by-step procedure that will assist in preventing a problem from escalating into a crisis situation. The previous tools can now be applied to assist you in gathering factual information for each of the steps.

1. *Prepare a problem statement.* Articulating a problem statement ensures that the underlying dynamics or causes of the problem are being explored, not a symptom of the problem.

2. *Obtain and interpret the facts.* The more information one has, the more accurate the solution will be. Interpreting data accurately also assists one in delineating the extent, severity, and projected impact that the problem discloses.

3. *State the desired objectives.* Objectives should be clearly understood and measurable. Once the problem is understood, as well as the underlying dynamics, objectives toward reaching a solution can be formulated.

4. *Generate alternatives utilizing both qualitative and quantitative analyses.* Quantitative factors to include may be items such as cost, error rates, and turn-around time. Qualitative factors may include impact on employee morale and employee resistance to change.

5. *Formulate criteria for evaluating alternative solutions; evaluate each alternative solution; then choose the best alternative solution.* Many analytical tools and activities can be used here.

6. *Develop an action plan.* As the action plan is being developed, trouble-shoot the solution so that one can build in flexibility "check points" in case unexpected variances should occur.

7. *Develop a plan for continuous quality improvement.* This includes immediate follow-up after implementation, as well as monitoring the desired outcomes. Communicate findings. Reevaluation is necessary and may mean going back to the drawing board . . . and that is okay!

Modified from Umiker, W. (1995). Decision making and problem solving by the busy professional. In H. Rowland & B. Rowland, *Nursing administration manual*. Vol. I. Rockville, MD: Aspen Publishers.

**Management Principles**

## ☀ Management Spotlight

### PLAY DOWN YOURSELF AND BUILD UP OTHERS

- Be a cheerleader. Point out strengths of others; give praise for doing things correctly.
- Play the game in such a way that one's presence makes others perform at a higher level.

From Pritchett, P. (1997). *The team member handbook for teamwork.* Dallas: Pritchett & Associates.

interviewer's skill. The content is what transpires during the interview.

1. *Make arrangements for employee input.* The employee should be given advance notice of the meeting and a copy of the evaluation form. The employee should be asked to prepare a list of objectives, contributions to the workplace, and goals for career development. In addition, employees should be asked to be prepared to share with the manager specific requests for support from management. Fig. 3-13 depicts an example of an employee self-evaluation form that can be used for multilevel positions and various work settings.

2. *Review the employee's personnel file.* These records should include the position description and standards of performance, continuing education and attendance records, commendations and special recognition, and incident reporting and records of counseling or disciplinary actions.

3. *Review the departmental objectives* or anticipated revisions of policies that may affect the employee.

4. *Provide the employee with a copy of the following* (make this material available to the employee well in advance of the interview):

- Position description
- Report of last performance appraisal

**Employee Self- Evaluation Preparation for**
**Annual Performance Appraisal**

NAME:                              POSITION:                              DATE:

Please complete for the following period of _____; Return to Director NLT _____.

1.   List professional goals / accomplishments achieved during the past year:

2.   Projects worked / completed and subsequent outcomes: (Describe the impact that the initiative had on the organization as a whole, not just your department)

3.   Annual required education completed (please attach documentation)

     CPR / BLS : _____
     Infect Cntrl: _____
     Fire/Safety: _____
     Competencies:

     Other:

4.   Educational programs attended or taught during the past year:   Total number of CE hours:

5.   Certification (s) and / or membership in professional organization(s):

6.   Civic / Community involvement during the past year:

7.   Future, long-term goals:

8.   Leadership activities and contributions to the organization  to be better positioned in a managed environment:

9.   Specific goals / projects for upcoming year:      What is keeping you from reaching your fullest potential?

10.  What changes in procedures, cost-containment techniques, or unit improvements originated from your suggestions?

11.  What do you think has been your most valuable contribution to the organization:

12.  What can management do to help you achieve your goals or to meet your needs?

**Thank you for your time in assisting me to provide you a meaningful performance appraisal interview.**

**Fig. 3-13**   Sample Employee Self-Evaluation Form.

- Current appraisal form to be used
- Employee preparation list or self-evaluation form (see Fig. 3-13)

5. *Discuss the employee's performance* with other observers to include other interfacing disciplines.

6. *Prepare an agenda* (set time and date) and *formulate key remarks.* Select the exact words (rehearse if necessary) to use for introductory statements, to state weaknesses and opportunities for improvement, and to confront defensiveness. Always try to "sandwich" criticism between two "slices" of praise. Employees usually get the point, and the defensiveness is manageable. Anticipate problem scenarios. Be prepared to cite specific examples to illustrate your points to offer specific examples of performance improvement opportunities. In addition, give employees illustrations of how to achieve advance or model ratings in the future.

### Handling the Performance Appraisal Process[*]

- *Maintain objectivity.* Each factor should be rated separately and independently. In other words, the halo effect must be avoided (e.g., the superb technical skills of an employee cause a manager to forget that the person never is on time). The reverse halo effect (the poor aspects of an employee's interpersonal skills overshadow the fact that the person always volunteers to help when a crisis occurs) must also be avoided.
- *Include supporting comments.* Comments should be included for each factor rated. For example, if the employee is marked "unsatisfactory" on attendance, a notation should be inserted that supports this conclusion (e.g., the employee was absent ten days during the year under evaluation, all of them single days off). These comments provide supporting documentation for the conclusion, and they demonstrate to the employee that the rating has an objective basis.

[*] From Henry K. (1995). *Nursing administration and law manual.* In H. Rowland & B. Rowland, *Nursing administration manual,* Vol. I. Rockville, MD: Aspen Publishers.

- *Discuss the evaluation with employee.* The evaluation should be reviewed with the employee, point by point. Evaluations serve little purpose and provide no notice if they are completed and filed without being communicated fully to the employee.
- *Respond to employee disagreement.* If employees disagree with a rating or opinion, or with any of the comments or conclusions, the ratings and conclusions should be double-checked, even if this means further investigation to determine the accuracy of the individual's comments.
- *Sign and date the evaluation.* When the final evaluation is ready, and again after it has been discussed with the employee, the employee should sign the form to acknowledge its review. Also, the manager should ensure that the date of the evaluation and the date of the employee's signature are included. These may become pertinent to a challenged supervisory action.
- *Cope with employee's refusal to sign.* If an employee refuses to sign an evaluation, the manager should not force the issue. It should be explained that signing does not indicate the employee's agreement with the evaluation's contents but is an acknowledgment that the employee saw it, reviewed it, and received a copy. If the employee continues to refuse to sign, the facts of refusal and the evaluation's review with the individual on a particular date should be noted. It may also be wise to have a second manager sign as a witness to the fact that the evaluation was reviewed with the employee (if applicable). A copy should then be given to the individual.
- *Review all evaluations periodically.* Managers should review all evaluations completed during a specific time period to determine whether any common problems appear to be surfacing. For example, if all employees, or a significant number of them, have been rated unsatisfactory on reporting in by the required hour or when they are sick, or on completing their nursing care plans, this is a signal that additional group notice or review of the applicable policies, standards, and expectations may be necessary before further enforcement attempts are made through disciplinary action.

Management Principles

- *Follow up on problem areas.* Where an assessment discloses unsatisfactory areas of performance, conduct, or absenteeism/tardiness, it should be identified for the employee what has to be done to correct the problem and a date by when the employee should do it. Resources that may be of help to the employees may also be identified.

## THE DISCIPLINE PROCESS[*]

All managers must occasionally handle disciplinary problems. When faced with this situation, the manager should:

### Know . . .

- What the unacceptable behavior is (past and present).
- Any mitigating circumstances.
- The scope of managerial authority.
- The policies of the organization.
- Union contract provisions relating to discipline.
- The way in which similar offenses have been handled in the department.

### Assume . . .

- That the employee may not know what is expected.
- That the employee wants to be a good performer.
- That he or she or others may be partly to blame.

### Act . . .

- Do it yourself. Do not delegate this task.
- Get all the information you can before you act.
- Consult with your superior and/or the personnel department.
- Act quickly once you have the facts.
- Practice progressive discipline.
- Act consistently and fairly. Do not discriminate.

---

[*] From Umiker, W. (1995). Management skills for the new health care supervisor. In H. Rowland, & B. Rowland, *Nursing administration manual.* Rockville, MD: Aspen Publishers.

- Discipline the employee in private.
- Select the action appropriate for the seriousness of the offense and the number of times you have addressed this problem before with the employee.
- Keep cool. Do not take any action when upset.
- Be tentative about pronouncing the sentence until you have checked with your superior and/or the personnel department.
- Document—document—document.
- Monitor the employee's performance carefully after the disciplinary action.

Levels of infractions and disciplinary action are described in Table 3-2 and Figs. 3-14 and 3-15.

## CONFLICT MANAGEMENT

Management issues usually emphasize conflict resolution; however, it is essential for a leader to understand that conflict is also a process. Since conflict is a process, it can be assumed that the potential exists to thwart a conflict or at least prevent escalation of one. Dove (1998) outlined seven stages of conflict to assist managers to effectively identify potential conflict situations:

1. *Antecedent conditions* set the stage for potential conflict. According to Dove, there are also nine characteristics of social relationships that precipitate conflict:
   - Ambiguous jurisdiction (roles and boundaries unclear)
   - Conflict of interest
   - Communication barriers
   - Dependent groups
   - Degree of differentiation (greater complexity and size of organization increases potential for conflict)
   - Association-related conflict (informal relationships between groups)
   - Need for consensus
   - Behavior regulation mechanisms (policies and procedures)
   - Prior unresolved conflict

**Table 3-2**   Infraction Levels and Their Management

| Class | Typical Infraction | Offense | Discipline |
|---|---|---|---|
| **Class I: Minor infractions** | Unsatisfactory quality or quantity of work | First | Oral warning |
| | Discourtesy to patient, staff members, or coworkers | Second | Written warning |
| | Lateness | Third | 1-day suspension |
| | Absenteeism | Fourth | 3-day suspension |
| **Class II: More serious infractions** | Unavailability when scheduled for work | First | Written warning |
| | Performance of personal work on hospital time | Second | 3-day suspension |
| | Violation of smoking, safety, fire, or emergency regulations | Third | Discharge |
| | Unauthorized absence | | |
| **Class III: Still more serious infractions** | Insubordination | First | Written warning |
| | Negligence | Second | Discharge |
| | Falsification of records, reports, or information | | |
| | Improper release of confidential or privileged information | | |
| | Sexual harassment | | |
| **Class IV: Most serious infractions** | Absence without notice for 3 consecutive days | First | Discharge |
| | Fighting on the job | | |
| | Theft or dishonesty | | |
| | Intoxication or use of alcohol or drugs on premises | | |
| | Willful damage to hospital property | | |

From Umiker, W. (1995). *Management skills for the new health care supervisor.* In H. Rowland & B. Rowland, *Nursing administration manual,* Vol. I. Rockville, MD: Aspen Publishers.

**FORMAL REPRIMAND**

| | |
|---|---|
| Employee's Name | Date |
| Job Classification | Department |

I. Problem: (Specify aspects of problem, dates, time, witnesses, pertinent information.)

II. Problem Results In:   (Policy, waste, safety, morale, quality of service.)

III. Corrective Employee Action:   (Specify what the employee is expected to do to improve.)

IV. Time to Improve:   (Some problems can be corrected immediately and others cannot. Indicate deadline for expected improvement.)

If problem continues, more severe disciplinary action may result.

Your signature on this form indicates that you have read and received a copy of it. Your signature does not indicate agreement with its content. If you disagree, you have five (5) days to file a grievance.

| | |
|---|---|
| Employee Signature | Date |
| Supervisor Signature | Date |

DISTRIBUTION:   WHITE - PERSONNEL   ●   CANARY - EMPLOYEE   ●   PINK - SUPERVISOR

Courtesy of Good Samaritan Medical Center, Phoenix, Arizona.

**Fig. 3-14**   Sample Counseling Documentation.
(Courtesy Good Samaritan Medical Center, Phoenix, AZ.)

2. *Perceived conflict* occurs when antecedent conditions remain unresolved; usually mistrust and anger are underlying issues.
3. *Felt conflict* involves feelings and attitudes; individuals are either judged or threatened by others; fosters mistrust.

Management Principles

EASTERN NEW MEXICO
MEDICAL CENTER

**Progressive Counseling and Development Plan**

Date: ______________

**DOCUMENTED VERBAL COUNSELING** ___

**WRITTEN STATEMENT** ___ **PROBATIONARY STATUS** ___ **# DAYS** ___

**SUSPENSION** ___ **# DAYS** ___ **TERMINATION** ___ **EFFECTIVE DATE** ___

**Employee's Printed Name:** ______________________________

**Manager's Signature:** ______________________ **Date:** ______________

**Employee's Signature:** ______________________ **Date:** ______________

1. Write the specific violation, concern or poor work habit.

2. Write why this a concern to you. Identify the impact on the work place or group.

3. Discuss and write down the employee's reason(s) why this problem occurred.

4. Identify the specific action(s) to be taken and by whom to resolve the situation.

5. Write down the date, time, and methods for follow-up with employee.

If termination, Human Resources must sign below prior to the completion of the action.
**Human Resource Representative Signature:** ______________________________

8270-001 12/93 **Copy 1- PERSONNEL FILE** **Copy 2- EMPLOYEE'S COPY** **Copy 3- MANAGER'S COPY**

**Fig. 3-15** Sample Disciplinary Action Form.
(Courtesy Eastern New Mexico Medical Center, Roswell, NM.)

4. *Depersonalized conflict* is evident when the behavior of groups creates a problem.
5. *Manifest behavior* occurs when groups exhibit overt behavior.
6. *Resolved or suppressed* happens when rationality remains an issue.
7. *Resolution aftermath* results in positive or negative feelings, depending on outcomes.

**Causes of Conflict**

Conflicts cause individuals to let emotions and behavior impede productivity; work does not get done efficiently and mistakes are made. Swansburg (1990) further asserts that defiant behavior is commonly seen in the workplace as an attempt to create conflict for the manager. He describes three types of individuals who challenge authority through obstinate and intransigent behavior (both verbal and nonverbal).

Three versions of the defier are:

- *Competitive bombers.* These are chronically angry people who scowl and mutter complaints under their breath and to others. Competitive defiers can be aggressive underminers who plan deliberate assaults. They complain about unfair and terrible working conditions and lousy schedules.

  If these people do not elicit a response from the manager, they sulk and complain to win the pity of peers, physicians, and even higher management.

- *Martyred accomodators.* These defiers use malicious obedience. They work and cooperate, but they do it with mocking complaints to enlist the support of others.

- *Avoiders.* These individuals avoid commitment and participation; they are reluctant to respond and often do not. As changes occur, they avoid participating, if possible, or may do so only temporarily.

Other causes of conflict include stress, space, physician authority, personal values and goals, organizational change, and new technology.

- *Stress.* Confrontation, disagreements, and anger are evident when stress develops from unfulfilled expectations. This situation leads to poor team interaction, job dissatisfaction, inefficiency, and insensitive patient care.

- *Space.* If working conditions are crowded and logistics are such that the flow of traffic (other team members, physicians, visitors) impede efficiency, frustration ensues.

- *Physician authority.* Authority is a source of conflict for many nurses. Nurses want to be more independent and feel that they contribute to the plan of care for a patient. Physicians differ in their treatment of nurses.

Management Principles

Certain physician behaviors diminish self-worth, causing nurses to become angry, lose confidence, and avoid communication.

- *Personal values and goals.* Incompatible perceptions or activities create conflict. Increasingly, ethics-related issues are surfacing in healthcare settings.
- *Miscellaneous.* Change causes conflict, which in turn impedes change. Both job and personal problems affect work performance and conflict. New technology, such as computers, can cause conflict or additional stress in the workplace.

### Possible Solutions

Dove (1998) suggests six strategies to use for resolving conflict:

1. *Compromising or negotiating.* Each party must commit to equal sacrifice for compromise to be perceived as a win-win situation.
2. *Competing.* Losing groups may feel angry and frustrated. Information is a tactic often used to take the advantage.
3. *Accommodating.* This approach is the opposite of competition. One individual or group sacrifices its belief or goal for others, often resulting in a "you owe me" attitude.
4. *Smoothing.* This tactic is designed to reduce the emotional component of the conflict by focusing on areas of agreement rather than opposition. Unfortunately, the root issue is seldom addressed.
5. *Avoiding.* This approach involves choosing to ignore a conflict, even though both parties recognize that it exists. This method can be used for trivial conflicts or when conflict requires that resolution be obtained without interference.
6. *Collaboration.* This tactic attempts to use assertive cooperation to resolve conflict. It focuses on depersonalization to allow both groups to employ problem-solving techniques.

Marrelli (1997) published the following manager's tips for resolving conflicts:

- Know that conflict is inevitable and that not all conflict is destructive.
- Always work toward helping staff members settle differences themselves.
- View yourself not as a parent but as an objective observer only.
- Validate that you will not take sides.
- Be objective.
- Support harmony and resolution.
- Verbalize that staff members need to talk to each other and that you trust their problem-solving skills.
- Listen with understanding, not judgment.
- Clarify the issue only when necessary.
- Do not criticize or deny feelings such as anger or fear.
- Focus on maintaining the relationship between the conflicting parties.
- Create a problem-solving atmosphere.
- Offer your space for a limited time for the discussion when appropriate.
- Be able to identify a chronically complaining employee. This is important because such behavior can contribute to a depressing tone for the entire work environment.

Two key elements are necessary for successful conflict resolution—trust and rationally. Additional essentials are open communication, quality circles to decrease stress and increase motivation, assertiveness training, and frequent positive feedback.

## BIBLIOGRAPHY

American Hospital Association. (1995). Patient representation in contemporary health care. In H. Rowland & B. Rowland, *Nursing administration manual.* Rockville, MD: Aspen Publishers.

Dove, M. A. (1998). Conflict: Process and resolution. *Nursing Management, 29*(4), 30–33.

Drucker, P. (1995). *Managing in a time of change.* New York: Truman Tally Books/Dutton.

Golightly, C. (1995). Creative problem solving for healthcare professionals. In H. Rowland & B. Rowland, *Nursing administration manual.* Rockville, MD: Aspen Publishers.

Katz, J., & Green, E. (1997). *Managing quality: A guide to system-wide performance management in health care* (2nd ed.). St. Louis: Mosby.

Marrelli, T. M. (1997). *The nurse manager's survival guide: Practical answers to everyday problems.* St. Louis: Mosby.

Rowland, H., & Rowland, B. (1995). *Nursing administration manual* (Vol. 1). Rockville, MD: Aspen Publishers.

Rowland, H., & Rowland, B. (1995). *Nursing administration manual* (Vol. 2). Rockville, MD: Aspen Publishers.

Schroeder, P. (1994). *Improving quality and performance: Concepts, programs, and techniques.* St. Louis: Mosby.

Swansburg, R. (1990). *Management and leadership for nurse managers.* Boston: Jones & Bartlett.

Umiker, W. (1995). Decision making and problem solving by the busy professional. In H. Rowland & B. Rowland, *Nursing administration manual.* Rockville, MD: Aspen Publishers.

Umiker, W. (1995). Management skills for the new health care supervisor. In H. Rowland & B. Rowland, *Nursing administration manual.* Rockville, MD: Aspen Publishers.

# Part Two

# Financial Responsibilities

# Chapter 4

# Quality and Productivity

*M*aking *resources productive is the specific job of management, as distinct from other jobs of the manager: entrepreneurship and administration. It is only managers— not nature or laws of economics or governments—that make resources productive.*

*Peter Drucker*

## IMPROVING PRODUCTIVITY

Healthcare changes have forced healthcare providers to maintain value to sustain a viable organization. Value simply means providing quality care cost effectively. Goals cannot be set without considering the implementation costs. Productivity targets cannot be met if perceived quality is compromised. Therefore quality and productivity must both be managed together, not as separate entities.

### Quality

Quality describes the attributes or characteristics of an element—the degree of excellence something possesses, its superiority.

**119**

## Productivity

Productivity is the action of producing abundantly. It is the creation of economic value, the production of goods and services.

According to Kirk (1988a), in order for quality and productivity to be compatible and to be accomplished, healthcare providers and managers need to question and overcome to survive financially:

*Myth 1:* The more quality that is wanted, the more it will cost.

*Myth 2:* There is no such thing as too much quality.

*Myth 3:* Quantity leads to quality. More is better.

Therefore healthcare providers must be able to communicate quality in terms of appropriateness, effectiveness, efficacy, and efficiency. Fundamentally, quality must be measured in terms of whether a standard has been met.

Standards are usually communicated in relationship to care, performance, or resources (Kirk, 1988a):

- *Care:* Identify what is to be accomplished.
- *Performance:* Describe specific care provider actions.
- *Resources:* Target staff hours required to achieve the predetermined care standard.

Define the acceptable level of quality, then budget for the resources (labor, supplies, equipment) that will enable you to maintain or exceed the targeted standard of care. Box 4-1 presents suggestions on specific approaches to improve productivity as viewed by one author.

> **BOX 4-1**
>
> ## Approaches to Improving Productivity
>
> Following are some suggestions on specific approaches to improving productivity:
>
> - *Measure of nursing productivity.* Develop a measure of nursing productivity based on nursing outcomes through the following steps:
>   1. Define nursing outcomes and determine how these should be measured. Include the following:
>      —Health status
>      —Patient knowledge
>      —Patient satisfaction (measured indirectly and directly)
>   2. Define patient-oriented goals based on these nursing outcomes.
>   3. Measure the extent to which these goals are achieved (this is a measure of nursing quality).
>   4. Utilize this nursing quality measure as a part of a nursing productivity measure (the other part being efficiency—use of resources to deliver the quality).
> - *Role definition.* Improve the role definition of the nurse at all levels, from director of nursing service to staff nurse, and do it both in leadership and clinical areas.
>   —Utilize personnel at levels consistent with their competence and preparation.
>   —Provide management training for nurses at the master's level and through inservice education.
>   —Involve the nurse in the development of his or her own role.
>   —Study the disparity between nursing education and nursing practice, and determine how to reduce or eliminate it.
> - *Participative management.* Encourage experimentation with and research into participative nursing management.
> - *Incentives.* Develop and use quality, financial, and other incentives for both individuals and the institution. Determine through research the extent to which incentives can affect productivity.
> - *Technological factors.* Investigate the interrelationship of various factors that affect nursing productivity (e.g., the relationship between nursing care organization [team, functional, primary] and facility design).
> - *Mechanization and automation.* Develop a model for nursing productivity that will accomplish the following:

*Continued*

---

**BOX 4-1—cont'd**

—Utilize quantified outputs and inputs.
—Fit into a model of health services evaluation.
—Utilize as inputs nursing personnel, facilities, equipment, supplies, etc.
—Provide output measures of patient health status, knowledge, and satisfaction.

From A review and evaluation of nursing productivity (1995). DHEW Pub. No. (HRA)77-15. In H. Rowland & B. Rowland, *Nursing administration manual.* Gaithersburg, MD: Aspen Publishers.

---

**BOX 4-2**

### WHEN DOES PRODUCTIVITY INCREASE?

**Productivity Increases**

| *When the Hours Worked* | *And the Units of Service* |
| --- | --- |
| Decrease | Stay the same |
| Decrease faster | Decrease |
| Stay the same | Increase |
| Increase | Increase faster |

From Kirk, R. (1988b). *Healthcare quality and productivity: Practical management tools.* Rockville, MD: Aspen Publishers.

---

To optimize both productivity and quality, standards must be communicated in relationship to efficiency and effectiveness—in other words, *doing things right* and *doing the right things.* Basically, productivity improves in specific situations (Box 4-2).

### Service Units

The unit of service (UOS) or modality is the common denominator that enables the identification and measurement of activities in terms of both quality and quantity (Table 4-1).

According to Rowland and Rowland (1995a-b), formal researchers have identified factors that should be considered for optimal organizational productivity. These are:

**Table 4-1** Examples of Service Units or Modalities

| Department | Unit of Service/ Modality | Time Measure |
|---|---|---|
| Emergency | Total visits | Hours per visit |
| Physical Therapy | Treatments | Hours per treatment |
| Food Service | Patient or cafeteria meals | Hours per meal |
| | Dietitian visits | Hours per visit |
| Surgery | Operations and procedures | Hours per operation |
| Laboratory | Tests | CAP units |
| Housekeeping | Square footage | Weighted square footage |
| Nursing (inpatient) | Patient day | Hours per patient day (HPPD) |

From Kirk, R. (1988a). *Healthcare staffing and budgeting: Practical management tools.* Rockville, MD: Aspen Publishers.

- Employee compensation tied to performance and sharing of productivity gains
- Participation of employee decisions affecting their related job and environment
- Job enrichment to include a sense of challenges, variety, and shared governance and involvement in the total organization
- Adequate safety conditions, pay, fringe benefits, and working conditions
- Simplification and access to channels of communication and authority
- Resources and tools available to facilitate work effectiveness
- Improvement of work efficiencies and subsequent reduction of frustration
- Greater attention to opportunities for meeting the needs of employees
- Allowance for flexibility in relation to the type of incentive and authority patterns

## Management Spotlight

### STRENGTHEN THE LEADER THROUGH GOOD FOLLOWERSHIP

Leaders cannot take a team to high performance if the team members are lousy followers. Followship involves people who lead themselves, are highly committed to do what is needed to do, without being told.

From Pritchett, P. (1997). *The team member handbook for teamwork.* Dallas: Pritchett & Associates.

Being cognizant of these factors should allow a manager to attempt to assess the department's strengths and weaknesses in relationship to prioritized opportunities for improvement.

Many authors agree that leadership is the key to optimal outcomes in quality and productivity. In addition, leaders are alert to the external environment and seek out new opportunities and inspire others to cooperate in the design and implementation of the new opportunities. This truth is depicted in the following prose by Witter Bynener (Kirk, 1988).

. . . But of a good leader, who talks little when his work is done, his aim fulfilled, they will say; "We did it ourselves."

### Key Result Areas

*The Pareto principle* holds that 20% of our time and effort produces 80% of the results. Proactive managers and administrators identify the most important 20% of their responsibilities, those that optimize quality within cost and productivity constraints, and subsequently direct 80% of their energies into achieving those goals.

Many authors agree that the success of achieving successful quality and productivity results directly relates to effective

**BOX 4-3**

## HOW TO BRING OUT THE BEST IN YOUR STAFF

1. Hire the right people for the job.
2. Share responsibility for growth, education, and development.
   • Be a mentor; groom and prepare staff and invest in them.
   • Beware; they'll appreciate while the equipment depreciates.
   • Have "winner" role models do the training/development.
3. Negotiate expectations and responsibilities.
   • Note where discipline will come into play.
   • Spell out rewards and how to earn them.
     —Pay for performance with management incentives.
     —Promote for performance (clinical and management).
     —Have clear, fair, competency-based job opportunities.
     —Give frequent recognition.
4. Involve employees in setting and deciding how to achieve goals.
   • Don't just talk about participative management . . . do it!
     —Use team building and group work to solve problems.
     —Give "scoop" first hand . . . so staff feels in on things.
     —Stay in touch, wander, and talk to corporate entrepreneurs who can fix a problem before it becomes one.
   • Show staff members their opinions matter. Act on their suggestions:
     —Quality circles
     —Hot lines
     —Meetings with management
     —Suggestion committees

From Kirk, R. (1988b). *Healthcare quality and productivity: Practical management tools.* Rockville, MD: Aspen Publishers.

leadership and the skill of actively involving staff members in this process (Box 4-3).

## WORK SIMPLIFICATION AND STREAMLINING

Many organizations are faced with workload dilemmas, such as funding for additional care hours. Proactive managers find positive ways to streamline the workload and prevent compromise of quality standards. Kirk (1988a) suggests involving the staff in solutions as much as possible, for example:

- Review each activity and procedure with the staff to evaluate whether efficiency could be improved.
- Redesign the method of giving change-of-shift reports (e.g., walking rounds). Use standardized, systematic report formats.
- Evaluate current documentation systems and begin to benchmark against best practices (e.g., focus charting, automation).
- Encourage staff to polish their organizational and time management skills. Productivity becomes a major problem when individuals cannot carry their own workload. Staff must be skilled in setting priorities.
- Encourage teamwork.
- Constantly communicate in a variety of methods. Communicate quality and productivity issues as a standing agenda item at staff meetings. Elicit solutions from staff when possible.
- Choose preceptors wisely. New employees, as well as managers, will benefit from having positive role models doing the orientation for new employees.
- Utilize various other individuals to augment your staff to do specific tasks within a department. Retired volunteers and high school volunteers are commonly seen in healthcare organizations.
- Develop policies and procedures that reflect efficiency. Ensure that staff have working knowledge of them. Involve selected individuals to craft the needed policies for a department.
- Use management information systems within the organization to analyze financial data and select cost-containment priorities and opportunities. Benchmark against best practices elsewhere in the region.
- Schedule patients and activities by using a systematic method that works.

- Avoid duplicate endeavors. Collaborate with other departments to streamline the workload.
- Use task forces to get specific tasks accomplished. If one group works well and enjoys the responsibility, give them the option to do another project.
- Evaluate organizational structure. Ensure that policies support a cost-contained but quality-based productivity system.
- Consistently delegate to the lowest scope of practice when possible (saves time and money).
- Explore the feasibility of having employees use pocket pagers or portable telephones to increase their mobility, thus improving productivity.
- Explore all new ideas!

## WHY FINANCE IS IMPORTANT

*No margin; no mission.*
  *Sister Irene Krause, Daughters of Charity Healthcare System*

- Healthcare is a service and a business.
- Financial issues affect everyone.
- Managed care and contracted care are growing.
- Cost management is vital to the viability and success of an organization.
- Organizations must manage within cost constraints; utilization and resource management are key essentials.

According to Richard Clark (1998), CEO (chief executive officer) of the Healthcare Financial Management Association, increased volume is not the answer to success. The key essential is prudent utilization of resources. He further states that to ensure success, healthcare systems must demonstrate the following attributes:
  - Integration: both horizontal and vertical
  - Market power: geographical coverage

- Risk-taking ability
- Low-cost approach
- Measurable quality

In addition, Clark (1998) asserts that the CFO (chief financial officer) and the CNO (chief nursing officer) share *similar competencies*. They are to:

- Recognize the mission (margin relationship)
- Benchmark against industry standards
- Interface to become part of the whole system
- Develop innovative strategies
- Communicate/develop/coach staff

Clark gives further insight into the paradigm shift facing healthcare organizations. He suggests that successful organizations believe and live the following concepts:

- Do not solve problems. Solving problems = investing in weaknesses; seeking opportunities = banking on the network.
- Doing exactly the right thing is far more productive than doing the same thing better.
- The new economy plays right into human strengths; the innovative, original, and imaginative all soar in value.

As innovative models and service delivery systems are created, the following objectives should be included to ensure cost containment without compromising quality (Burns, 1998):

1. Focus on high-quality patient care and patient satisfaction.
2. Ensure appropriate clinical expertise.
3. Enhance staff satisfaction.
4. Improve service to referring physicians.
5. Build on teamwork and accountability.
6. Continually advance knowledge.
7. Deliver clinical effectiveness and operational efficiency.
8. Support infrastructure efficiency and evaluation systems.
9. Have sustainable goals.

Innovative models and emerging service delivery systems involve consolidation. According to Burns (1998), associate professor of healthcare systems at The Wharton School in

Philadelphia, the *rationale for consolidation* of healthcare entities includes:

- Economies of scale (bigger is cheaper—lower cost and lower price)
- Economies of scale (breadth is better—one-stop shopping)
- Expansion of the service delivery network (allows greater access)

Burns further declares that successful organizations achieve optimal economies of scale by centralization of management, purchasing and materials management, and other key service functions. Hospitals have not done this well.

## TYPES OF ORGANIZATIONAL BUDGETING

Budgeting is a logical way for any business organization to control its costs. *Budget* is defined as a quantitative expression of a plan of action that results in attaining efficiency and effectiveness. *Efficiency* is the relationship between input and output. *Effectiveness* is the relationship between an organization's output and its objectives.

The following are basic budget methods commonly used in organizations and companies that deal with issues of efficiency and productivity (Strasen, 1987). These principles are subsequently used at the divisional and departmental levels within the organization.

1. Incremental budgeting
2. Planning, programming, and budgeting (PPB)
3. Management by objectives (MBO)
4. Zero-based budgeting (ZBB)

### Incremental Budgeting

In developing an incremental budget, the previous year's actuals are used as the starting point. Amounts are then added for inflation and new programs. Budgeting is done by responsibility or cost center. This method is easy to do. The weaknesses of this type of budget are that (1) one must assume that last year's amount was correct, and (2) it focuses only on input. Minimal, if any, evaluation regarding benefits is done (American College of Healthcare Executives Tutorial, 1998).

### Planning, Programming, and Budgeting

PPB is an approach introduced by President Lyndon Johnson in 1965 as a formal method of budgeting in the federal government. According to Strasen (1987), the most important budgeting principle that comes from PPB is the development of objectives to determine which programs and/or services are financially supported by the organization. The steps in the PPB process are:

- Development of departmental goals and objectives
- Evaluation of each program and service to meet those objectives, including a cost-benefit analysis
- Exploration of alternative programs and services
- Development of the budget based on an analysis of the alternative programs/services to meet the objectives and financial parameters established

### Management by Objectives

MBO was originated by Peter Drucker in the 1950s. It was introduced into the federal government in 1973, when the MBO process became more popular. MBO is very similar to PPB, but it does not require the extensive financial analysis of alternative services to accomplish the organizational's objectives.

### Zero-Based Budgeting

ZBB was developed by Peter Phyrr at Texas Instruments in the 1970s. This method emphasizes management's responsibility for planning, budgeting, operationalizing, and evaluating the organization's resources. ZBB requires an analysis of alternative programs and services on three levels: minimum, current, and improvement objective levels. It requires ranking program and service priorities and systematically allocating resources (Strasen, 1987).

The major objectives (Strasen, 1987) for planning a budget are to:

- Force managers to analyze the organization's activities for appropriateness
- Direct management's attention toward the future
- Enable management to proactively identify problems or opportunities for improvement to provide timely interventions
- Remind managers of the actions to which commitment was made
- Reinforce managers' motivation to work diligently to achieve the organizational objectives
- Provide a reference point for control reporting

The length of budget periods used are generally referred to as fixed or rolling. According to Cleverly (1992), a fixed budget is more frequently used in healthcare institutions. This type of budget covers a defined period of time, usually 1 year. This approach contrasts with a rolling budget, in which the budget is extended on a frequent basis. For example, for every new month, another month would be added so that the budget is always projecting a total of 12 months.

The rolling budget offers significant advantages; however, it also requires more time and effort. Healthcare organizations that use this type of budgeting often enjoy success and viability (Cleverly, 1992). Cleverly asserts that the major advantages of the rolling budget are:

- More realistic forecasts, which should improve management planning and control
- Equalization of the workload of budget development over the entire year
- Improved familiarity and understanding of budgets by department managers

## Flexible or Forecast Budgeting

A flexible budget is a more sophisticated method than typical forecast budgeting and is commonly used by healthcare facilities that are experienced in the budgetary process (Cleverly, 1992). A *flexible budget* is one that adjusts targeted levels of costs for changes in volume. A *forecast budget,* in contrast, makes no formal differentiation in the allowed budget between these two levels.

## FINANCE AND ASSETS MANAGEMENT

Because of the importance of financial viability to almost every aspect of the organization's operations, competent financial management is necessary for effective and efficient hospital operations. The basic concepts of healthcare finance are usually found in three academic disciplines: financial accounting, managerial accounting, and financial management.

- *Financial accounting* involves the basic accounting functions of data entry, transaction analysis, and preparation and interpretation of financial statements for internal managers and external stakeholders.
- *Managerial accounting* targets the internal uses of accounting information for decision making. Managerial accounting techniques include cost identification and cost/volume/profit models. This approach should provide information to improve the efficiency and effectiveness of the use of economic resources.
- *Financial management* focuses primarily on assets management with an emphasis on cash-flow analysis, including working capital, capital structure composition, risk and cost of various amounts of debt and equity sources, capital budgeting process, time, value of money techniques, and financial feasibility studies.

## BUDGET REVIEW QUESTIONS

The following budget review questions are sample questions that each manager would ask, within the individual's scope of responsibility, and organizational level, to optimally develop a projected budget. These questions are not all-inclusive. Keep in mind the strategic plan, goals, and prioritized strategies for the proposed budget year.

1. What opportunities are there for increased volume, and to what extent are they reflected in your proposed operating budgets?

2. What opportunities are there for resource management (reduced use of patient charge items such as laboratory tests, x-rays, drugs, etc.) in your department, and to what extent are they reflected in your proposed operating budgets?

3. Does your proposed staffing reflect work redesign initiatives? If so, what is the impact on your customers (patients, physicians, other hospital departments), and have they been included or considered in evaluation of the proposed redesign?

4. How do you plan to increase your ability to flex with volume and/or redesign work to reflect the level of activity indicated in the major volume assumptions? To what extent can staff "stretch" to meet the volume increase between baseline and moderate growth budgets?

5. What cost reduction strategies have you incorporated into your operating budgets?

6. What support is required to accomplish the objectives incorporated into your proposed operating budgets?

7. How does your department(s) compare to industry standards?

8. What opportunities not reflected in the proposed operating budgets do you plan to continue to evaluate?

9. How would you complete the following statement? *This department could significantly improve its performance/efficiency/effectiveness if only* _____
_____.

10. Regarding your capital budget requests, explain the strategic or nondiscretionary nature of the request(s) and the degree to which it impacts your proposed operating budgets.

## PRESENTER PREPARATION GUIDE

The presenter should be prepared to review background material, as well as have detailed information available, to support the proposed operating budgets and capital requests. Background and other materials should be provided to the budget council or finance committee before the scheduled presentation date (Box 4-4).

### Glossary and Formulas for Labor Budgeting (Fig. 4-1 and Box 4-5)

$$\text{Quality standards} + \text{Labor hours needed to meet} = \text{Unit of service standard quality standards}$$

The standard care hours required per *UOS* is a predetermined decision with a specific allocation of time, for example,

---

**BOX 4-4**

### SAMPLE OUTLINE FOR PRESENTING PROPOSED BUDGET TO FINANCE COMMITTEE OR BUDGET COUNCIL FOR APPROVAL*

**Background Material**
Function(s)
Scope of services
   Description
   Hours/days of operation
Staffing/organization chart
History/trends
Strategic initiatives (including organizational impact analysis, resource requirements, and other support requirements)
   Volume
   Resource consumption
   Cost management
   Cross-departmental/cross-functional initiatives
   Work redesign/value-added analysis
Industry comparisons (particularly best practices/benchmarking)

---

*As defined by the healthcare organization.

## BOX 4-4—cont'd

**Supporting Detail**
Volume
Opportunities to increase business
Opportunities to reduce resource consumption
Trend analysis
Major customers
Inpatient and outpatient mix
Revenues
Average revenues per-unit-of-service trend analysis
Charge master revisions (revenue neutral)
Staffing
FTEs by position
Coverage
Flexibility
Part-time/full-time mix
72-hour positions
Value added by position/hours covered
Supplies
Relation to units of service
Relation to average charge per unit of service
Cost avoidance measures
Alternate items/vendors
Reusable versus disposable
Unit of issue
Product expiration monitoring
Inventory versus nonstock items
Other nonsalary expenses
Have details available (not just historical trends)
Nondiscretionary
Explain necessity/risk of not acquiring
Discretionary
Explain value added by expenditures
Cost/benefit analysis
Capital
Nondiscretionary
Explain necessity/risk of not acquiring
Strategic
Explain value added by expenditure
Cost/benefit analysis

---

**Calculating Standards
Using Retrospective Classification Data**

*The goal is to target average volume and average acuity so that one can budget the
appropriate personnel resources needed to provide anticipated services.*

| Specific Department Modality/UOS | Modalities/UOS Completed | | Required Hours per Modality/UOS* | | Staffing Hours Required |
|---|---|---|---|---|---|
| UOS #1 - 30 minutes | 1000 | × | 0.5 | = | 500 |
| UOS #2 - 45 minutes | 1000 | × | 0.75 | = | 750 |
| UOS #3 - 1 hour | 1000 | × | 1.0 | = | 1000 |
| UOS #4 - 1.5 hours | 1000 | × | 1.5 | = | 1500 |
| UOS #5 - 2 hours | 1000 | × | 2.0 | = | 2000 |
| UOS #6 - 3 hours | 1000 | × | 3.0 | = | 3000 |
| **Totals:** | **6,000** | | | | **8,750** |

| Total Staff Hours Required | ÷ | Total Modalities | = | Average Required Labor **Hours Per Modality** Based on Acuity & Volume |
|---|---|---|---|---|
| 8,750 | | 6,000 | | 1.5 Hours/Modality or Unit of Service |

**Fig. 4-1** Calculating Standards Using Retrospective Classification Data.

(From Kirk, R. [1988]. *Healthcare staffing and budgeting: Practical management tools.* Rockville, MD: Aspen Publishers.)

0.5 nursing hours per patient modality (visit, exercise session, or patient day).

## Supportive Information for Developing a Department Standard (Kirk, 1988a)

1. Measure the labor hours consumed by patient care and other service task documents:
   • Hours per modality/UOS (visit, procedure, test, day)
   • Relative value units (of a predetermined number of minutes) per unit of service
2. Track the above data on logs or reports:
   • Provides information about changing patterns (seasonal, marketshare) of resource labor hour consumption
   • Provides retrospective data:
     —Modality intensity (acuity)
     —Modalities per discharge patient
3. Identify the volume and diagnostic distribution of current patients/clients:

**BOX 4-5**

## Glossary and Formulas for Labor Budgeting

**Definitions Used in Budgeting for Labor**

*FTE* = Full-time equivalent, refers to a full-time position, usually 40 hours per week

*Work week* = 40 hours per week, usually 5 days

*Workday* = 8-hour shift

*Shift* = 8 hours

*Work year* = 2080 hours

*0.2 FTE* = 8 hours per week

*1.4 FTE* = 7 shifts per week

**Calculations Used in Budgeting for Labor**

*Average occupancy* = Number of beds × Percent occupancy

*Hours per patient day × Average census* = Total nursing hours for the unit

*Total hours per day ÷ by 8 hours* = Number of FTEs for 24 hours.

*Hours per patient day (HPPD)* = Average hours of care per patient for 24 hours

*Direct care* = Delivery of direct patient care

*Indirect care* = Administration, education, clerical, and other support personnel

*Direct and indirect hours* = Hours worked and paid for

*Nonproductive hours (NPH)* = Hours paid for and not worked, holidays, vacations, etc.

*Total FTEs* = All paid hours in a week divided by 40

*Percent staff per shift × Total FTEs* = FTEs per shift

*Percent staff ratio* = Professional to nonprofessional

*Number of hours worked per hours in work week* = FTE (8 hours ÷ 40 = 0.2 FTE)

From Nelson, E. M. (1987). Budget. In B. Rutkowski, ed., *Managing for productivity in nursing.* Rockville, MD: Aspen Publishers.

- Helps managers to rank diagnoses to identify the utilization patterns of department services by both volume and intensity.
- Helps managers identify the intensity (acuity) measures to update or validate patient care and other service needs concurrently.

## Full-Time Equivalents (FTEs) (Fig. 4-2 and Table 4-2)

- *Total adjusted FTE* is the sum of the flexible (direct), fixed, and nonproductive FTEs. It then becomes the *position control* (i.e., total number of FTEs that can be hired).
- *HPW,* or hours per workload unit, is the target that reflects nursing care required in 24 hours for each unit of work. This includes only productive or worked time.
- *HHPD,* or hours per patient day, is the number of paid hours divided by the patient days.
- *Budgeted hours per UOS:* multiply the direct or productive FTEs by the annual FTE worked hours (2080) to determine the direct care/service hours. Divide the direct care/service hours by the projected (or actual) total UOSs.

> EXAMPLE: 21.5 Productive FTEs × 2080 Annual hours = 44,720 direct care hours
>
> 44,720 Direct care hours ÷ 6721 UOSs = 6.7 Budgeted hours per UOS

- To determine *acuity,* divide the workload by the census.

> EXAMPLE: 24 ÷ 18 = 1.33 (acuity)

## Table 4-2 FTEs

*1.0 FTE* is a position for one full-time employee or two or more part-time employees.

*1.0 FTE* is equal to 2080 hours annually.

*0.4 FTE* accounts for 4 days in a 2-week pay period and is the standard relief for a 7-day-per-week position. (The 1.0 FTE works five 8-hour shifts/week, and the 0.4 FTE works to cover for the full-time person's 2 days off).

**Full-Time and Part-Time FTEs** *(During 2-Week Period)*

| Days Worked | Hours Worked | Annual Hours | % of 1.0 FTE |
| --- | --- | --- | --- |
| 10 | 80 | 2080 | 1.0 |
| 8 | 64 | 1664 | 0.8 |
| 6 | 48 | 1248 | 0.6 |
| 5 | 40 | 1040 | 0.5 |
| 4 | 32 | 832 | 0.4 |
| 2 | 16 | 416 | 0.2 |

## PART I—STAFFING PATTERN

| | 7–3 | 3–11 | 11–7 | Total |
|---|---|---|---|---|
| Head nurse[†] | 1 | | | 1 |
| Registered nurse | 4 | 3 | 3 | 10 |
| Nurse's aides | 2 | 1 | | 3 |
| Ward clerk[†] | 1 | 1 | | 2 |

[†]Head nurse and ward clerk indirect.

Multiply each category by 1.4 to find total FTEs in each category.

Multiply total FTEs by 2,080 to obtain hours worked.

Use average percentage for hospital NPH (5% is used here) to calculate replacement hours.

Use average percentage for unit overtime.

## PART II—STAFFING SCHEDULE

The annual staffing schedule based on the above daily staffing pattern should look like this:

| Classification | FTEs | Hours Worked |
|---|---|---|
| Head nurse | 1.0 | 2,080 |
| Staff nurses | 14.0 | 29,120 |
| Nurse's aides | 4.2 | 8,736 |
| Ward clerks | 2.8 | 5,824 |
| Totals | 22.0 | 45,760 |
| Replacement | 1.1 | 2,233 |
| Overtime | .5 | 1,040 |
| Budgeted | 23.6 | 49,033 |

If census varies on a daily basis, the same method can be used to develop variable staffing guides for direct care. This can be helpful in developing scheduling patterns. A good patient classification and staffing system will provide this type of information.

**Fig. 4-2** One Approach to Calculating FTEs.

(From Nelson, E.M. [1987]. Budget. In H. Rowland & B. Rowland [Eds.]. *Nursing administration manual.* Rockville, MD: Aspen Publishers.)

## Acuity- and Volume-Based Staffing Budget

1. Average daily census × Acuity × Hours per workload = Total productive hours/24 hours
2. Total productive hours × Time unit (usually total calendar days in year) = Total productive hours for flexible caregivers required for the specified time unit (usually annual)
3. Total annual productive hours ÷ 2080 (hours worked for 1.0 FTE) = Total flex productive FTEs
4. Next, add the number of fixed FTEs. Finally, add the number of nonproductive hours/FTEs according to the individual institution's guidelines.
5. Determine the labor expense per UOS.

EXAMPLE

Predetermined values:

   Units of service (UOS): 6721

   Average daily census (ADC): 18.4 (UOS ÷ 365 days/yr)

   Acuity: 1.16

   Hours per workload (HPW): 5.7

$$\text{ADC (18.5)} \times \text{Acuity (1.16)} \times \text{HPW (5.7)} =$$
$$\text{122.32 Productive hours/24 hours}$$

$$\text{122.3} \times \text{Time unit (365 days/year)} =$$
$$\frac{\text{4639.5 (total productive hours for flex caregivers)}}{\text{2080 (annual hours worked for 1.0 FTE)}}$$
$$= \text{21.5 FTEs (productive) caregivers required}$$

   21.5 FTEs (productive)
   +3.4 FTEs (fixed)
   ──────────────
   24.9 FTEs TOTAL

## Budget Targets as Productivity Measures
(Kirk, 1988b)

The following are miscellaneous formulas often used in analyzing and projecting productivity and workload management information.

### *Actual total HPM*

| Total hours paid | ÷ | Actual modalities | = | Actual total HPM |
|---|---|---|---|---|
| 1640 | ÷ | 2000 | = | 0.8 |
| Target hours | − Actual hours | ÷ Target hours | = | % over (under) budget target |
| 1.0 | − 0.8 | ÷ 1.0 | = | (20%) |

NOTE: Example is a 4-week period.

### *Actual direct HPM*

| Total hours paid | − Nonproductive hours paid | − Fixed hours paid | = | Actual direct hours paid |
|---|---|---|---|---|
| 1640 | − 160 | − 480 | = | 1000 |
| | | (3 fixed × 160) | | |
| Direct hours paid | ÷ | Actual modalities | = | Acutal direct HMP |
| 1000 | ÷ | 2000 | = | 0.5 |
| Target HPM | − Actual direct | ÷ Target HPM | = | % over (under) budget target |
| 1.0 | − 0.5 | ÷ 1.0 | = | (50%) |

NOTE: Example is a 4-week period.

### *Actual total salary costs per modality*

| Total actual salary costs | ÷ | Actual period modalities | = | Actual total salary costs per modality |
|---|---|---|---|---|
| $20,000 | ÷ | 960 | = | $20.83 |
| Target costs | − Actual costs | ÷ Target costs | = | % over (under) budget target |
| $21.50 | − $20.83 | ÷ $21.50 | = | (3%) |

NOTE: Example is a 4-week period.

### Percentage rate of absenteeism

$$\frac{\text{Total absences in period}}{\text{(Total annual FTE} \times \text{Workdays in period)}} \times 100 = \text{Absenteeism (\%)}$$

$$\frac{15 \text{ absences in 4 weeks}}{(26.7^* \times 20[4 \text{ weeks} \times 5 \text{ days}]) = 534} \times 100 = \quad 2.8\%$$

NOTE: Example is a 4-week period.

*Given information

### FTE per occupied bed

| Total hospital FTE | ÷ | Average daily census (actual) | = | FTE per occupied bed |
|---|---|---|---|---|
| 550.0 | ÷ | 160 | = | 3.4 |

### Ratio of hours worked to hours paid

Total hours worked ÷ Total hours paid[‡] = Hours worked-to-paid ratio

| 3872[†] | ÷ | 4207 | = 92% of worked hours are productive |
|---|---|---|---|

[†]Data available from payroll system or department.
NOTE: Example is a 4-week period.

### Percentage of filled positions

Number of FTE hired ÷ Total authorized positions = % Filled positions

| 24.3 | ÷ | 26.7 | = | 91% |
|---|---|---|---|---|

### Overtime rate

Overtime hours paid ÷ Total hours paid = Overtime rate

| 125 | ÷ | 4640 | = | 2.7% |
|---|---|---|---|---|

*Average direct care hours per modality*

Ideally, direct hours per modality (HPM) are time studied and valued directly. If you want to know the HPM currently budgeted for in your department, use this formula:

Direct FTE × 2080 ÷ Projected modalities = Average direct care HPM

| 5.3 | × 2080 ÷ | 11,000 | = | 1.0 |

## Workload Distribution (Fig. 4-3)

1. Determine productive hours required for 24 hours.
2. Determine percentage of total staff for each shift.
3. Calculate FTEs required for each shift based on first two assumptions:

Productive hours/24 hours × Shift staffing percent ÷ Hours in one shift

4. Determine skill mix for each shift based on the number of FTEs allowed for each shift.

---

**Cost Center:** _____ **FY:** _____

**Current Classification Activity:**

| Patient Type | ADC | Relative Value | Average Workload |
|---|---|---|---|
| 1 | 6.3 | 0.4 | 2.5 |
| 2 | 15.0 | 1.0 | 15.0 |
| 3 | 6.4 | 2.0 | 12.8 |
| 4 | 1.0 | 4.4 | 4.4 |
| Total: | 28.7 | | 34.7 |

Workload __34.7__ ÷ ADC __28.7__ = Average Acuity: __1.21__

**Projected Workload:**

Patient Days: __11, 133__ ÷ 365 = ADC: __30.5__

ADC: __30.5__ × Average Acuity: __1.21__ = Workload: __36.9__

---

**Fig. 4-3**  Sample Current and Projected Workload.

(From Finkler, S. [1992]. *Budget concepts for nurse managers.* Philadelphia: WB Saunders.)

EXAMPLE: Workload distribution (continuing from previous calculations)

$$\frac{\text{122.3 Productive hours}}{24} \times \begin{array}{l} \text{D } 0.38 = 46.5 \div 8 = \quad 5.8 \quad 6.0 \\ \\ \text{E } 0.37 = 45.3 \div 8 = \quad 5.7 \quad 6.0 \\ \\ \text{N } 0.25 = 30.6 \div 8 = \quad 3.8 \quad 3.0 \end{array}$$

TOTAL            1.0        15.3 Budget        15.0 Actual

Skill mix may be 50% registered nurses (RNs) and 50% certified nurse assistants (CNAs); therefore on day shift, three RNs and three CNAs would be scheduled based on assumed volume and acuity. If volume or acuity changes, then these FTEs would "flex" to reflect changes.

Percent occupancy = Census ÷ Beds available × 100

Average length of stay (ALOS) = Patient days in given time period ÷ Number of discharges in same time period

### Patient Classification/Acuity

1. Utilizing the institution's patient classification, identify the relative value points for each patient type.
2. For each patient type, determine the ADC. Multiply by the relative value point to determine the average workload for each patient type.
3. Total workload ÷ Total ADC = Average acuity

### Calculating Break-Even Points

- *Break-even point* is the point at which the revenues equal the expenses.
- *Contribution margin* is the amount of revenue left after the direct costs of providing the service are subtracted.

EXAMPLE (Marrelli, 1997):

| | |
|---|---|
| Monthly fixed costs: | $10,000 |
| Revenue per visit: | $100 |
| Direct cost per visit: | $50 |
| Contribution margin: | $50 |

Contribution margin = Revenue per visit − Direct cost per visit

$$\$100 - \$50 = \$50$$

Therefore the break-even point (point at which next unit of service's contribution margin is considered profit) would be:

$$\$10,000 \div \$50 = 200 \text{ visits}$$

- *Census-related break-even point* is the level of census required to cover the fixed costs of the minimum staffing level.

EXAMPLE (Strasen, 1987):

| Medical/Surgical Unit | Standard: HPPD 5.0 | Minimum Staffing: 2 RNs per shift |
|---|---|---|
| 7-3 Shift | 3-11 Shift | 11-7 Shift |
| 2 RNs = 16 hours | 2 RNs = 16 hours | 2 RNs = 16 hours |
| 1 NM = <u>5.7 hours</u> | | |
| 21.7 hours | | |

21.7 Hours + 16 Hours + 16 Hours = 53.7 Hours

53.7 ÷ 5 HPPD = 10.7 Patients (minimum census)

## BUDGET PLANNING, MONITORING, AND CONTROL (KIRK, 1988b)

- Know your product. Identify and validate the hours per unit of service. Know costs for services at varying levels of quality.
- Identify costs first, then direct efforts toward decreasing costs while maintaining quality; increasing efficiencies while improving quality; and reducing hours per UOS while maintaining quality.
- Work simplification ideas to diminish workload if hours per UOS are lower than what is ideally required.
- Use the standard hours/UOS to budget, monitor, and evaluate flexible budgeting.
- Adjust staffing to workload.
- Develop an annual productivity plan for each department that includes expected volume, FTEs, labor and nonlabor expense per UOS, staffing parameters based on volume, and projected nonproductive time.

- Keep ongoing profile of absenteeism and communicate results to staff.
- Plan and organize for the most effective utilization of skilled labor.
- Cost out staff training and development: Set targets for orientation expenses, and work out reward systems to help with expenses for classes and continuing education.
- Monitor overtime critically. Find out why it is occurring and correct excesses. Is it an individual productivity problem? Does it require approval?
- Maintain and build flexibility into staffing to help meet budget and classification targets.
- Determine staff reduction plans. Ensure that policies reflect activities of staff reductions. Work with staff for contingency plans for low volume. If rightsizing the organization, communicate clearly and as far in advance as possible.

### Variance Analysis: Comparing Actual Performance to Classified Need and Budgeted Expectations

All 3 hours per UOS targets must be considered in order to maintain an effective monitoring and evaluation system:

1. *Actual hours provided:* Is staffing within budget restraints?
2. *Budgeted hours financed:* Is department adequately budgeted to meet patient care needs?
3. *Classified hours needed:* Is acuity level congruent with care provided?

Figs. 4-4 through 4-7 present samples of variance reporting.

### Cost-Effective Ways to Survive Prospective Payment Systems

*Prospective payment system (PPS)* is defined as payment based on a predetermined price for any particular category of patient (e.g., a particular diagnosis related group [DRG]), as opposed to reimbursement based on the costs of care provided to the patient.

## Example
### Budget/Staffing Worksheet

Cost Center: _____6020_____                                      PPE: ___9/20___

| | Date | 9/7 | 9/8 | 9/9 | 9/10 | 9/11 | 9/12 | 9/13 | 9/14 | 9/15 |
|---|---|---|---|---|---|---|---|---|---|---|
| DAYS | C/Ac | 19/1.14 | 19/1.13 | 23/1.18 | 23/1.24 | 24/1.19 | 20/1.15 | 22/1.11 | 19/1.03 | 22/.92 |
| | A/R | 5/6.0 | 5/5.3 | 7/7.1 | 7/7.5 | 7/6.8 | 6/6.0 | 6/6.3 | 5/5.1 | 5/4.6 |
| EVENINGS | C/Ac | 18/1.13 | 20/1.18 | 21/1.24 | 22/1.19 | 20/1.15 | 21/1.11 | 20/1.03 | 19/.92 | 21/1.04 |
| | A/R | 4.5/5.1 | 5/5.9 | 6/6.5 | 6/6.5 | 6/5.7 | 6/5.9 | 5/5.2 | 4/4.5 | 5/5.3 |
| NIGHTS | C/Ac | 19/1.13 | 22/1.18 | 22/1.24 | 22/1.19 | 21.1.15 | 22/1.11 | 19/1.03 | 19/.92 | 21/1.04 |
| | A/R | 3/3.6 | 4/4.5 | 4/4.3 | 4/4.5 | 4/4.0 | 4/4.2 | 3/3.3 | 3/3.0 | 4/3.8 |
| | | | | | | | | | | |
| | Flex Total | 12.5 | 14 | 17 | 17 | 17 | 16 | 14 | 12 | 14 |
| | NM | 0 | 1 | 1 | 1 | 1 | 1 | 0 | 0 | 1 |
| | CC | 0 | 0 | 0 | 1 | 0 | 0 | 0 | 0 | 0 |
| | Day US | 1 | 1 | 1 | 1 | 1 | 1 | 1 | 1 | 1 |
| | Even US | .5 | 1 | .5 | 1 | 1 | 1 | .5 | .5 | 1 |
| | Fixed Total | 1.5 | 3 | 2.5 | 4 | 3 | 3 | 1.5 | 1.5 | 3 |
| | Total | 14 | 17 | 19.5 | 21 | 20 | 19 | 15.5 | 13.5 | 17 |
| | MN CEN | 19 | 22 | 22 | 22 | 19 | 21 | 19 | 19 | 20 |
| | OBS | 0 | 0 | 0 | 0 | 2 | 1 | 0 | 0 | 1 |
| | BUD FTE | 17.59 | 20.37 | 20.37 | 20.37 | 19.45 | 20.37 | 17.59 | 17.59 | 19.45 |
| | VAR | −3.59 | −3.37 | +.87 | +.63 | +.55 | −1.37 | −2.09 | −4.09 | −2.45 |

**Legend:**                                      **Comments:**
C/Ac = Census/Acuity
A/R = Actual Staff/Recommended
NM = Nurse Manager
CC = Clinical Coordinator
US = Unit Secretary
MN CEN = Midnight Census
OBS = Observation Patients
VAR = Variance Btwn Flex Total
     FTE & Budgeted FTE

**Fig. 4.4, *A*** Sample and Form of Budget/Staffing Worksheet.

*Continued*

# Example
## Budget/Staffing Worksheet

Cost Center: ____6020____     PPE: __9/20__

| | Date | | | | | | | |
|---|---|---|---|---|---|---|---|---|
| DAYS | C/Ac | | | | | | | |
| | A/R | | | | | | | |
| EVENINGS | C/Ac | | | | | | | |
| | A/R | | | | | | | |
| NIGHTS | C/Ac | | | | | | | |
| | A/R | | | | | | | |
| | | | | | | | | |
| | Flex Total | | | | | | | |
| | NM | | | | | | | |
| | CC | | | | | | | |
| | Day US | | | | | | | |
| | Even US | | | | | | | |
| | Fixed Total | | | | | | | |
| | Total | | | | | | | |
| | MN CEN | | | | | | | |
| | OBS | | | | | | | |
| | BUD FTE | | | | | | | |
| | VAR | | | | | | | |

**Legend:**
C/Ac = Census/Acuity
A/R = Actual Staff/Recommended
NM = Nurse Manager
CC = Clinical Coordinator
US = Unit Secretary
MN CEN = Midnight Census
OBS = Observation Patients
VAR = Variance Btwn Flex Total
      FTE & Budgeted FTE

**Comments:**

**Fig. 4.4, *B*** Sample Blank Form.

**Example**
**Patient Care Services**
**Bi-Weekly FTE Analysis**

**Cost Center:** _6020_                                             **Pay Period** _9/7-9/20_

Units of Service:

_282_ MN Census                    _5_ Observation Census           _287_ Adjusted Total Census

Budgeted FTEs:

Productive Hours/Units of Service:     _6.445_ Flexed         _0.964_ Fixed

Calculations:  Flexed: _287 × 6.445 ÷ 80 = 23.12_
              Fixed: _287 × 0.964 ÷ 80 = 3.45_

Actual FTEs:                          Actual FTE Breakdown:

Regular Hours:  _1990.66_            Flex hours:    _1701.9_  = _21.27_  FTEs
OT Hours:       _37.7_              Fixed hours:   _326.46_  = _4.08_   FTEs
Holiday Hrs:    _—_                 Orientation:   _0_       = _0_      FTEs
                       Education:     _0_       = _0_      FTEs
Total:          _2028.36_           NonProd:       _333.4_   = _4.16_   FTEs

Variance/Explanation:

Flexed:     Budget Variance  _<1.85>_          Classified Recommendation:  _21.1_          Fixed Budget Variance:    _+.63_

**COMMENTS:**

*Continued*

**Fig. 4-5** Sample and Form of Patient Care Services Biweekly FTE Analysis.

**Patient Care Services**
**Bi-Weekly FTE Analysis**

**Cost Center:** _____

**Pay Period** _____

Units of Service:

_____ MN Census _____ Observation Census _____ Adjusted Total Census

Budgeted FTEs:

Productive Hours/Units of Service: _____ Flexed _____ Fixed

Calculations: Flexed: _____

Fixed: _____

Actual FTEs:

Actual FTE Breakdown:

| | | |
|---|---|---|
| Regular Hours: _____ | Flex hours: _____ = _____ | FTEs |
| OT Hours: _____ | Fixed hours: _____ = _____ | FTEs |
| Holiday Hrs: _____ | Orientation: _____ = _____ | FTEs |
| | Education: _____ = _____ | FTEs |
| Total: _____ | NonProd: _____ = _____ | FTEs |

Variance/Explanation:

Flexed _____ Budget Variance _____ Classified Recommendation: _____ Fixed Budget Variance: _____

**COMMENTS:**

**Fig. 4-5** Cont'd. Sample and Form of Patient Care Services Biweekly FTE Analysis.

**OVERTIME REPORT**

Unit: _____     Date: _____

PP Ending: _____

**Overtime Total:** _____

     Incremental: _____

     Mandatory Meeting: _____

     Inservices: _____

     Pre-Sched OT: _____

     Replacement: _____

     Holiday: _____

**Explanation for each category of OT:**

_____
_____
_____
_____
_____

**Plans to Decrease OT:**

_____
_____
_____
_____
_____

**Fig. 4-6**  Sample Form of Overtime Report.

Benefits of cost finding (Kirk, 1988b):

- If cost exceeds price, a department cannot be considered to be financially independent or successful in business.
- The use of costs as baseline information for costing care and services can lead to a change in the productivity of a department, such as generating increased revenue. It can also lead to a more equitable method of charging patients for services.

## Example
### Daily Productivity Worksheet

For Period ___9/7___ Through ___9/20___

Department _____

| | (1) | (2) | (2/1) | (from budget) | |
|---|---|---|---|---|---|
| Date | UOS | Total Hours Worked | Actual Hours/ UOS | Budgeted Prod.Hr./ UOS | VAR |
| 9/7 | 20 | 144 | 7.2 | 6.7 | +.5 |
| 9/8 | 19 | 120 | 6.3 | 6.7 | −.4 |
| | | | | | |
| | | | | | |
| | | | | | |
| | | | | | |
| | | | | | |
| | | | | | |
| | | | | | |
| | | | | | |
| | | | | | |
| | | | | | |
| | | | | | |
| | | | | | |
| | | | | | |
| | | | | | |
| | | | | | |
| | | | | | |
| | | | | | |
| | | | | | |
| | | | | | |
| | | | | | |

**Fig. 4-7, *A*** Sample Form of Daily Productivity Worksheet.

**Daily Productivity Worksheet**

For Period _____ Through _____

Department _____

| | (1) | (2) | (2/1) | (from budget) | |
|---|---|---|---|---|---|
| Date | UOS | Total Hours Worked | Actual Hours/ UOS | Budgeted Prod.Hr./ UOS | VAR |
| | | | | | |
| | | | | | |
| | | | | | |
| | | | | | |
| | | | | | |
| | | | | | |
| | | | | | |
| | | | | | |
| | | | | | |
| | | | | | |
| | | | | | |
| | | | | | |
| | | | | | |
| | | | | | |
| | | | | | |
| | | | | | |
| | | | | | |
| | | | | | |
| | | | | | |
| | | | | | |
| | | | | | |
| | | | | | |
| | | | | | |
| | | | | | |

**Fig. 4-7, *B*** Cont'd. Sample Blank Form.

- Identified costs provide useful information for program planning activities. Validated information gives credible support to decision making.
- Knowing the cost of providing a service is paramount for organizations to negotiate contracts in a managed care environment.

The following lists the responsibilities of the nurse administrator with respect to adapting to the PPS environment (Larson & Peters, 1995):

1. Communicate therapeutic effectiveness and cost-efficiency to staff nurses. Staff must become more involved to monitor, control, and reduce costs while maintaining or improving quality.
2. Collect and evaluate data on an organizational level. Empirical data should drive changes in practice to improve clinical outcomes.
3. Develop sophisticated clinical and staff development credentialing programs. Staff must be active in the multidisciplinary care planning of patients and must be knowledgeable to execute appropriate, independent, and professional judgments.
4. Master the economics of healthcare. Improved knowledge and skills in the business aspects of healthcare management will facilitate growth. Seek learning opportunities outside the industry; however, stay in tune with the healthcare industry's benchmarked "best practices" and standards.
5. Monitor measurements of productivity. Utilize quantified data from patient acuity rating systems to study use of personnel, supplies, and equipment. Revise and align staffing patterns as appropriate changes take place.

### Integration of Cost and Quality (Fig. 4-8)

There are six major areas that are critical to integrating cost evaluation and quality of care (Wilson, 1995):

1. Organizational support
2. Efficient systems

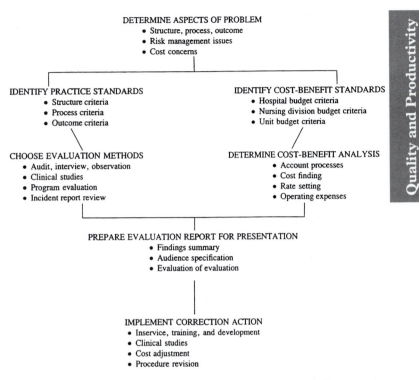

**DETERMINE ASPECTS OF PROBLEM**
- Structure, process, outcome
- Risk management issues
- Cost concerns

**IDENTIFY PRACTICE STANDARDS**
- Structure criteria
- Process criteria
- Outcome criteria

**IDENTIFY COST-BENEFIT STANDARDS**
- Hospital budget criteria
- Nursing division budget criteria
- Unit budget criteria

**CHOOSE EVALUATION METHODS**
- Audit, interview, observation
- Clinical studies
- Program evaluation
- Incident report review

**DETERMINE COST-BENEFIT ANALYSIS**
- Account processes
- Cost finding
- Rate setting
- Operating expenses

**PREPARE EVALUATION REPORT FOR PRESENTATION**
- Findings summary
- Audience specification
- Evaluation of evaluation

**IMPLEMENT CORRECTION ACTION**
- Inservice, training, and development
- Clinical studies
- Cost adjustment
- Procedure revision

**Fig. 4-8**   Integrating Cost and Quality Improvement Systems.

(From Wilson, C. [1995]. Strategies for monitoring the cost-quality of care. In H. Rowland & B. Rowland [Eds.] *Nursing administration manual.* Rockville, MD: Aspen Publishers.)

3. Multidisciplinary problem solving
4. Education
5. Access to information and financial data
6. Cost monitoring/cost analysis strategies

**Steps in Conducting a Cost Analysis** (Figs. 4-11, 4-12, and 4-13)

Whether to choose cost-benefit analysis (CBA) or cost-effectiveness analysis (CEA) depends on whether the purpose of the analysis is to compare the cost-benefit ratio of several programs or to compare the relative costs of several alternatives to achieve the same goal. The steps in conducting either

Date _____

Unit _____

Project/study title _____

Time period _____

POTENTIAL COST BENEFITS




COSTS

Total personnel costs _____

Supplies _____

CNRE charges _____

Total costs $ _____

Total time _____ hours

**Fig. 4-9**   Sample Cost-Benefit Analysis Summary/Quality Project or Study.

(Courtesy St. Michael Hospital, Milwaukee, WI.)

type of analysis can be delineated as follows (Larson & Peters, 1995):

1. Define the problem.
2. State the objective of the proposed program, practice change, or product.
3. Identify alternatives.
4. Define the perspective of the analysis. For example, does it represent costs and benefits to the patient or to employees? If it represents more than one viewpoint, each should be analyzed separately.
5. Analyze costs. Include both direct and indirect costs.
6. Evaluate benefits: in dollars for CBA, in effects for CEA.

**Fig. 4-10** Sample Cost-Benefit Worksheet for Project/study. (Courtesy St. Michael Hospital, Milwaukee, WI.)

Project/study title: _____

| Activity Parameters | Consultant | | DON | | CNS | | Head Nurse | | AHN/CC | | R.N. I | | R.N. II | | R.N. III | | Total |
|---|---|---|---|---|---|---|---|---|---|---|---|---|---|---|---|---|---|
| | Number | Time | Number | Time | Number | Time | Number | Time | Number | Time | Number | Time | Number | Time | Number | Time | |
| Preparation | | | | | | | | | | | | | | | | | |
| Consultation | | | | | | | | | | | | | | | | | |
| Meeting | | | | | | | | | | | | | | | | | |
| Collecting Data | | | | | | | | | | | | | | | | | |
| Data Analysis | | | | | | | | | | | | | | | | | |
| Dictation | | | | | | | | | | | | | | | | | |
| Reporting | | | | | | | | | | | | | | | | | |
| Other CNRE | | | | | | | | | | | | | | | | | |
| Supplies | | | | | | | | | | | | | | | | | |
| Xeroxing cost | | | | | | | | | | | | | | | | | |
| Additional | | | | | | | | | | | | | | | | | |

Personnel Utilized

Total Cost: $ _____

**PART I—RATING CRITICAL FACTORS**

**Purpose:** To involve staff leadership in determining the relative importance of critical factors in resource allocation.

**Instructions:** Assign a numerical rating to each and every factor by placing a check mark (✔) on the point along the scale that most closely expresses your opinion of the importance of the factor.

| CRITICAL FACTOR | RATING<br>Totally Unimportant<br>1 | 2 | 3 | 4 | 5 | 6 | 7 | 8 | 9 | Extremely Important<br>10 |
|---|---|---|---|---|---|---|---|---|---|---|
| 1. COMPATIBILITY WITH PURPOSE<br>The extent to which an activity or program is consistent with the mission and major goals of the institution. | | | | | | | | ✔ | | |
| 2. COMMUNITY SERVICE<br>The contribution of an activity or program to the institution's community obligation. | | | | | | ✔ | | | | |
| 3. PROFITABILITY<br>The contribution to profit or return on investment of an activity or program. | | | | | ✔ | | | | | |
| 4. FEASIBILITY<br>The ability of the institution to secure adequate resources to successfully implement a plan of action. | | | | | | | | | | ✔ |
| 5. QUALITY OF SERVICE<br>The extent to which an activity or program adds to the overall prestige and image of the institution. | | | | | | | | | | ✔ |

**PART II—RATING PROPOSALS USING CRITICAL FACTORS**

**Purpose:** To develop consensus on priorities by rating activity and program proposals in terms of critical factors.

**Instructions:** Assign a rating to each and every proposed activity or program by placing a check mark (✔) in the box that most closely expresses your opinion of the value of the proposal for each critical factor.

| Proposal | Compatibility with Purpose | | | Community Service | | | Profitability | | | Feasibility | | | Quality of Service | | |
|---|---|---|---|---|---|---|---|---|---|---|---|---|---|---|---|
| | Low | Mod | High | Low | Mod | High | Low | Mod | High | Low | Mod | High | Low | Mod | High |
| 1 | | | | | | | | | | | | | | | |
| 2 | | | | | | | | | | | | | | | |
| 3 | | | | | | | | | | | | | | | |
| 4 | | | | | | | | | | | | | | | |
| 5 | | | | | | | | | | | | | | | |
| 6 | | | | | | | | | | | | | | | |
| 7 | | | | | | | | | | | | | | | |
| 8 | | | | | | | | | | | | | | | |
| 9 | | | | | | | | | | | | | | | |

**Fig. 4-11** Sample Tool for Determining Critical Factors in Resource Allocation.

(From Dowd, R. [1988]. Participative decision making in strategic management of resources. In H. Rowland & B. rowland [Eds.]. *Nursing administration manual.* Rockville, MD: Aspen Publishers.)

7. Determine the present value of any future costs and benefits by calculating a discount. This is called discounting:

$$\text{Present value} = \text{Future value} \div (1 + \text{Interest rate})^{\text{interval in years}}$$

8. Analyze uncertainties. Substitute different values from within the range of possible values for costs and ben-

**Instructions:** Use the following codes in preparing the report:

1 = indicates that a sample has been reviewed
2 = reported only quarterly or yearly
3 = records will automatically be reviewed by department/committee or peers
NA = not available
\* = see NARRATIVE ANALYSIS for conclusion

| INDICATORS | JAN | FEB | MAR | APR | MAY | JUN | JUL | AUG | SEPT | OCT | NOV | DEC |
|---|---|---|---|---|---|---|---|---|---|---|---|---|
| **VOLUME INDICATORS** | | | | | | | | | | | | |
| Total numbers of patients | | | | | | | | | | | | |
| Total occupancy rate (%) | | | | | | | | | | | | |
| Average daily census | | | | | | | | | | | | |
| Total average length of stay (LOS) | | | | | | | | | | | | |
| Number of codes | | | | | | | | | | | | |
| **QUALITY/APPROPRIATENESS INDICATORS** | | | | | | | | | | | | |
| **General** | | | | | | | | | | | | |
| Number of incident reports | | | | | | | | | | | | |
| Custodial | | | | | | | | | | | | |
| Professional | | | | | | | | | | | | |
| Medication errors | | | | | | | | | | | | |
| All other | | | | | | | | | | | | |
| Number of written patient/family complaints | | | | | | | | | | | | |
| Number of written physician/staff complaints | | | | | | | | | | | | |
| Patient satisfaction questionnaire results (%) | | | | | | | | | | | | |
| Registered nurse hours/patient day | | | | | | | | | | | | |
| Number of readmissions within 30 days | | | | | | | | | | | | |
| Number of times unable to reach physician after ___ attempts | | | | | | | | | | | | |
| Problems identified through routine record review | | | | | | | | | | | | |
| Report(s) of potential problems referred from other departments/sources | | | | | | | | | | | | |

*Continued*

**Fig. 4-12**  Sample Form of Nursing Service Trend Report: Quality Appropriateness Indicators.

(From Rowland, H., & Rowland, B. [1995]. Nursing administration manual. Rockville, MD: Aspen Publishers.)

efits calculated to determine whether changes in the values will alter the conclusions of the analysis. This is called a sensitivity analysis.

9. Address ethical issues (e.g., the appropriate distribution of limited resources in the population, the accessibility of programs and resources, the extent to which the analysis can be influenced by bias).

10. Interpret results.

*Cost-benefit analysis (CBA)* is a system to evaluate the worth of a product or program; it can compare two programs with different objectives (e.g., the new trach sets and new IV

| INDICATORS | JAN | FEB | MAR | APR | MAY | JUN | JUL | AUG | SEPT | OCT | NOV | DEC |
|---|---|---|---|---|---|---|---|---|---|---|---|---|
| **Outcome** | | | | | | | | | | | | |
| Number of patients misassigned to unit | | | | | | | | | | | | |
| Number of LOS $\leq$ 24 hours | | | | | | | | | | | | |
| Number of patients AMA/AWOL | | | | | | | | | | | | |
| Number of IV infiltrates | | | | | | | | | | | | |
|   Peripheral | | | | | | | | | | | | |
|   Central | | | | | | | | | | | | |
| Number of multiple attempts to draw blood | | | | | | | | | | | | |
|   Arterial | | | | | | | | | | | | |
|   Femoral | | | | | | | | | | | | |
| Mortality rate (%) | | | | | | | | | | | | |
| Survival rate on codes (%) | | | | | | | | | | | | |
| Infection rate (%) | | | | | | | | | | | | |
| Number of medication errors | | | | | | | | | | | | |
| Number of adverse reactions/complications | | | | | | | | | | | | |
|   Unit | | | | | | | | | | | | |
|   Unit | | | | | | | | | | | | |
|   Unit | | | | | | | | | | | | |
| Number of malpractice cases (nursing) | | | | | | | | | | | | |
| Inappropriate implementation of physician orders | | | | | | | | | | | | |
| **Documentation and Process** | | | | | | | | | | | | |
| Total number of charts with incomplete documentation | | | | | | | | | | | | |
|   Number/% incomplete admission referral forms | | | | | | | | | | | | |
|   Number/% patient assessments not completed within ___ hours | | | | | | | | | | | | |
|   Number/% care/treatment plans not completed within 24 hours | | | | | | | | | | | | |
|   Number/% patient/family teaching not performed prior to discharge | | | | | | | | | | | | |
|   Number/% discharge planning notes not including expected outcomes | | | | | | | | | | | | |
| Number of delays $\leq$ 1 hour in X-ray or laboratory | | | | | | | | | | | | |
| Number of unscheduled tests | | | | | | | | | | | | |
| Total number of transfers | | | | | | | | | | | | |
|   In-house | | | | | | | | | | | | |
|   Out of house | | | | | | | | | | | | |

**Fig. 4-12** Cont'd. Sample Form of Nursing Service Trend Report: Quality Appropriateness Indicators.

start kits). *Cost-effectiveness analysis (CEA)* is a system to compare the relative costs of two or more product alternatives with the same objective (e.g., two types of IV infusion pumps).

## Components of a Quality Management Program
(Marker, 1995)

- Description (setting and scope of services performed)
- Philosophy of quality management (QM)/definition of *quality*
- Objectives for accomplishment via quality assessment

**STEPS†**

1. **Identify program components to be evaluated.** Based on feedback from various data sources (i.e., the patient and family, monitoring results, and findings from QA studies), a clinical, administrative, or educational component of the program requiring further assessment is chosen for study.
2. **Describe the methodology to be used.** The information collection process is defined according to the program evaluation questions being asked. Decisions are made regarding the appropriateness of qualitative or quantitative methods and the use of specific data collection instruments. For example, if patient satisfaction data are desired, an interview format using a qualitative approach may be used.
3. **Analyze and report the findings.** The findings are assessed with regard to three major questions: (1) Is there

indeed a programmatic problem? (If not, the process ends here.) (2) Does the problem require corrective action? (3) Who needs to be informed and take responsibility for corrective action?
4. **Make recommendations to implement corrective action.** Provide detailed information gleaned from the evaluation process to the appropriate individuals as defined in step 3. This information will become the basis for decision making.
5. **Evaluate the impact of the corrective action.** In order to complete the evaluation process, it is essential to follow up on the decisions made. Was the information utilized to make positive changes in the QA program? Both quantitative and qualitative methods may be used in this final step. If it is determined that there was no decision made or that the decision made was ineffective, the blocks to change are identified and, if appropriate, the evaluation process is reinitiated (see step 1).

**OUTLINE OF PROPOSED QA STUDY‡**

STUDY TOPIC

STUDY SIZE AND TIME PERIOD

STUDY OBJECTIVE

DESCRIPTION OF STUDY TOPIC

☐ Diagnosis    ☐ Special Procedure    ☐ Surgical Procedure    ☐ Problem or Condition    ☐ Other

PATIENT IDENTIFICATION DATA

Age
☐ All ages
☐ Exclude pediatric
☐ Exclude geriatric
☐ Only between _____

Sex
☐ Both sexes
☐ Males only
☐ Females only

IDENTIFICATION DATA

☐ Original study
☐ Repeat study
   date(s) of prior study(ies) _____
☐ Medical study only
☐ Nursing study only
☐ Combined patient care study

Date: _____

**Fig. 4-13**   Sample Form: Assessment of a Specific Problem.

(From Pelletier, L. & Poster, C. [1988]. An overview of evaluation methodology for nursing QA. In H. Rowland & B. Rowland. Nursing administration manual. Rockville, MD: Aspen Publishers.)

- Scope of QM activities
- Discussion of important aspects of care and indicator development
- Responsibilities
- Structure of activities (including committee structure, persons involved, and use of quality teams)
- Integration/coordination of events (within service/department, between services and higher authority)

- Data analysis/corrective action planning/problem resolution approaches
- QM documentation (organized manual of data assessment tools)
- QM reporting/communication (monthly/quarterly basis)
- Evaluation of effectiveness (annual summation)

## Guiding Principles for Continuous Quality Improvement

The executives at one healthcare institution (Wesley Medical Center, Wichita, KS) developed the following philosophy to incorporate a value framework that encouraged teamwork, cooperation, involvement, and dedication to continuous improvement (Rowland & Rowland, 1995).

- *Place quality first.* We make the quality of our products and services our number one priority. We will strive to eliminate barriers, rework, and complexity in the belief that benefits to our patients, market share, and profitability will follow.
- *Focus on the customer.* We recognize that there are many internal and external customers of the medical center, and we will strive to meet their needs. We will identify opportunities for improvement by listening to the voice of the customer.
- *Recognize our people as our most valuable asset.* We respect the talents people bring to their jobs and believe that people want to do their best. We will focus on systems improvements.
- *Acknowledge physicians as partners, as well as customers.* We recognize the essential relationship between the medical center and the medical staff. We will involve physicians in the constant improvement of systems.
- *Become partners with suppliers committed to continuous improvement.* We believe the value of a product or service is measured by more than price alone. We will build mutually beneficial relationships with suppliers committed to quality improvement.
- *Manage through leadership.* We show the way by example. We will share our vision, enable others to act, and promote teamwork.

- *Encourage pride of workmanship.* We believe in creating an environment that allows people to take pride in their work. We will empower people to identify and remove barriers to quality.
- *Treat one another with trust and respect.* We respect the worth of every individual. We will continuously improve our working relationships based on this principle.
- *Value honesty, trustworthiness, and integrity.* We are dedicated to doing the best for all concerned. We will treat patients, other customers, and one another as we would wish to be treated, recognizing that how we act *is* the Wesley product.
- *Seek continuous improvement in all we do.* We understand that quality is ever evolving. We will strive for excellence.
- *Utilize statistical processes to monitor systems and identify opportunities for improvement.* We seek continuous improvement of the process through reduction of variation. We will use data to understand the process.
- *Cease reliance on inspection to achieve quality.* We recognize that we cannot effectively achieve quality through inspection alone. We will use inspection as one means for listening to the voice of the system.
- *Understand that defects come from processes, not people.* We believe that waste, rework, and inefficiencies originate in defective systems. We will encourage people to improve the process.
- *Support education and training.* We value the growth and development of people. We will invest in job training and encourage self-improvement.
- *Promote innovation.* We support creative thinking in the improvement of systems and development of services. We will pay particular attention to the ideas of those closest to the work.
- *Celebrate achievements.* We believe in the value of recognizing improvements. We will take time to celebrate successes.

**Outcomes-Based Practice: Why Change?** (Grady, 1995)
*Healthcare has changed*
- Healthcare is the second largest industry (higher expenditures than those for defense and education).

- Healthcare is estimated to represent approximately 14% of GNP.
- There are hundreds of drugs to prescribe and tests to order.
- Cost containment while maintaining or improving quality is a tremendous challenge.
- It is estimated that 10% of the population consumes 80% of the resources.
- Organizations have decreasing net margins and increasing consumer demands.

### Methods for cutting costs
- Shotgun (lay-offs; reduction of FTEs)
- Rifle (take out a layer of management)
- Reduce services (mergers)
- Reduce quality (not feasible)
- Increase volume (consolidation of service areas)
- Change production process (outcomes management, critical pathways, streamlining of efficiencies)

### Philosophies for change
- *Service line management* is a method of alignment of necessary services for a particular patient population.
- *Case management* is a system of health assessment, planning, service procurement, delivery coordination, and monitoring that meets the multiple service needs of the patient.
- *Outcomes management* is the utilization of outcomes assessment information to enhance clinical and financial quality through integration of exemplary practice and service.

### Tools for standardization
- Pathways (clinical, financial, patient education)
- Standing orders
- Protocols
- Guidelines
- Algorithms
- Standards

*Critical pathways*
- Practice guidelines (standards of practice) for multiple disciplines
- Never a final draft
- Represents scientifically based healthcare practices
- Allows for aggregate analysis of care experience
- Identification of high-risk subgroups

*Practice outcomes*
- Allow for revisions in practice, values, and standards
- Promote collaborative philosophy and practice
- Encourage advanced education (analytical tools)
- Foster research utilization
- Strengthen quality improvement efforts
- Increase peer consultation, collaboration
- Promote continuity of care, coordination of care, and appropriate resource utilization

*Types of variances*
- Patient
- System
- Practitioner

*Evaluation (measures of quality and efficiency)*
- Length of stay
- Cost savings
- Patient education/compliance/discharge needs
- Complication incidence
- Consumer satisfaction
- Expected outcomes

*Descriptive statistics*
- Categorization, rank ordering, numerical scoring
- Describe sample
- Condense and organize data
- Explore relationships
- Assess variability

*Inferential statistics*
- Statistical analyses

## OUTCOMES PROGRAMS (JUHN, 1996)
- Performance monitoring
  —Report cards
- Quality measurement
  —Benchmarking
  —Outlier detection
- Guidelines development
  —Standards
  —Care maps
  —Protocols
- Disease management
  —Data information
  —Decisions continuum
- Technology assessment
  —Cost-effectiveness analysis
- Patient-centered outcomes
  —Functional health status
  —Quality of life
  —Satisfaction

### Driving Forces
- Accountability
- Monitoring
- Measurement
- Science
- Technology
- Quality
- Cost

### Challenges
- Data and information systems (relevant, timely, usable)
- Linkage to process ("what" caused by which "how")

- Decision-support capability (patients, members, providers, purchasers)
- Patient-focused measures (ultimate decision-makers)

## OUTCOMES RESEARCH (JUHN, 1996)

Outcomes research relies on studies to determine which treatments are effective and which are not and to identify those providers who are performing well and those who could do better.

### Value

- Measurement of clinical performance
  —Assess variations
  —Establish benchmarks
  —Focus improvement data
- Oversight of medical care
  —Early detection of important deficiencies in care
- Consistent with core value of "providing care of superior quality"

### Key Dimensions

- *Outcomes* are those changes, either favorable or adverse, in the health status of persons, groups, or communities that can be attributed to prior or current care.
- *Risk factors* are elements that are causally related to the outcomes under study.
- *Risk adjustment* is a mathematical method designed to remove or reduce the effects of risk factors in studies in which the cases are not randomly assigned to different treatments (Table 4-3).
- *Data source* is the information source, which can affect a study's clinical credibility, influence perception of its validity, and determine its reliability and accuracy.

  Sample tools for identifying and tracking outcomes are presented in Figs. 4-12 through 4-15.

**Table 4-3** Sample Risk-Adjusted Outcomes Studies

| Condition of Procedure | Outcome Measures |
|---|---|
| 1. Perinatal care | Perinatal mortality |
| 2. Acute myocardial infarction | Survival |
| 3. CABG | Operative mortality |
| 4. Hysterectomy | Post-op wound infections |
| 5. Hospital patients | Mortality in hospital and within 1 year of discharge |

From: Juhn, P. I. (1996). *The art and science of outcomes assessment: The roles of data, information and decisions.* Oakland, CA: Kaiser Foundation Health Plan.

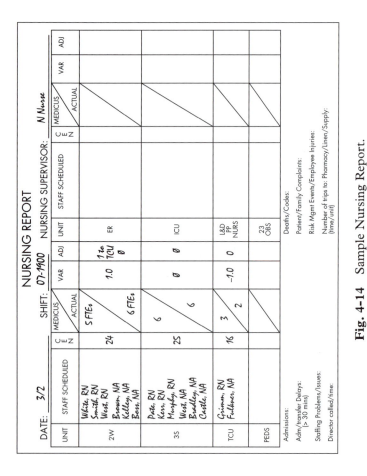

**Fig. 4-14** Sample Nursing Report.

Quality and Productivity

**EASTERN NEW MEXICO MEDICAL CENTER**
**END OF SHIFT REPORT - MEDICAL/SURGICAL**

Date:_____     Shift:_____     Unit:_____     Census:_____

| Admissions Room # | | Discharges Room # | | Surgeries Room # | | Emergency Procs Room # |
|---|---|---|---|---|---|---|
| | | | | | | |
| | | | | | | |
| | | | | | | |
| | | | | | | |
| | | | | | | Special Procedures |
| | | | | | | |
| | | | | | | |
| | | | Outstanding Employee: | | | |
| OBS Room # | | | Why: | | | |
| | | | Outstanding M.D.: | | | |
| | | | Why: | | | |

**Problems Related to:**

Bed Utilization_____
Physicians_____
Equipment/Supplies_____
Assignments/Co-Workers_____
Non-Productive Time_____
Other Departments_____
Pace/Workload:     Quiet     Steady     Busy     Very Busy     Short

**Report on Patients Who Develop (Include Room #):**
Decubitus Not Present on Admission_____
Decubitus Present On Admission That Worsens_____
Post-Op Respiratory Problems_____
Temp 101F or Greater_____
IV Phlebitis_____
IV Infiltrations_____
Post-Op Wound Infection_____
Blood Transfusion Errors_____
Number of Blood Transfusions_____
Complications with Epidurals or PCA Pumps_____
Hemorrhage_____
Colostomy Care_____

**Report Room Numbers for:**      Code Blue_____     Falls/Injuries_____
                                   DNR_____     Med Occurences_____
                                   Deaths_____     Outliers See Next Page____

| Transfers (Room #s) |
| Another Facility_____ |
| CCS_____ |
| Room Changes_____ |

Significant Events/Concerns/Comments_____
_____
_____

Signature(s):_____

**Fig. 4-15**   Sample End-of-Shift Report.

## PUTTING OUTCOMES MANAGEMENT INTO PRACTICE

One method of introducing practice outcomes management is to develop a multidisciplinary *clinical practice committee or council* within an organization (Fig. 4-16). Box 4-6 depicts the committee's conceptual framework and goals. In addition, it shows how one service area can use the committee to strengthen the independent professional accountability of its members.

**STANDARDS OF CLINICAL PRACTICE**

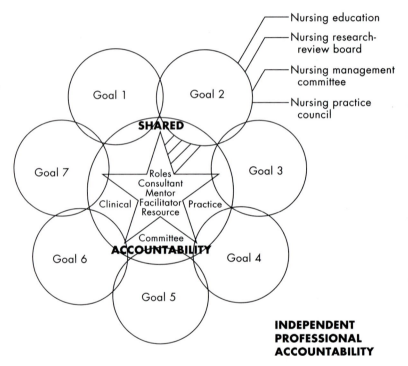

**Fig. 4-16** The clinical practice model depicts the conceptual framework in which a multidisciplinary committee can provide collaborative practice guidance, as well as strengthen individual practice accountability. The committee shares accountability by bench marking against practice standards and providing structure and resources. However, the care provider, within limits, then becomes accountable for implementation of the standards.

---

**BOX 4-6**

## CLINICAL PRACTICE COUNCIL

PURPOSE: To provide hospital-wide leadership and guidance in the promotion of quality clinical practice through educational programs, research, clinical protocols, and collaborative practice.

*Goal 1:* Decrease inconsistencies between the facility's standards of practice and professional performance.

*Goal 2:* Standardize credentialing in accordance with regulatory guidelines.

*Goal 3:* Influence changes in the healthcare system by promoting and expanding opportunities for (nursing) research and applying the findings to practice and decision making.

*Goal 4:* Guide departmental practice councils (or policy and procedure committee) in the development and attainment of practice standards.

*Goal 5:* Provide guidance for the development of a patient education program for the institution.

*Goal 6:* Strengthen the communication network and foster collaboration between practice and education.

*Goal 7:* Promote quality in standardizing education programs or service delivery systems by encompassing assessment, planning, implementation, and evaluation processes.

---

## SPECTACULAR CUSTOMER SERVICE
(BOX 4-7 AND *ACTION TIPS* BOX)

The two broad dimensions of customer service are the following:

- *Procedural dimension.* This aspect is related to the customer's awareness of how an organization or service delivery should be performed. The customer's perceptions of how systems operate and of the skill level of personnel are continuous challenges that healthcare providers face in an effort to exceed expectations.
- *Personal dimension.* This area encompasses each individual differently and plays out in attitudes, behaviors, and interpersonal relationships and skills. An example is what Disney's management staff describes as a "magic

**BOX 4-7**

# Spectacular Customer Service

**Customer Service: Procedural Dimension**

1. *Timing.* What are service delivery standards? Do customers wait long periods of time to have needs met or perceived service delivered?

2. *Flow.* How do departments and personnel interface with each other? Does the service provided flow seamlessly, or is it fragmented, choppy, and frustrating for the customer?

3. *Accommodation.* How flexible are the processes to meet special requests by customers? Are there indicators in place to measure this area of service?

4. *Anticipation.* How well are the customers' needs anticipated. Do customers have to request services that should be automatic or routine?

5. *Communication.* How does one know if communication is accurate and timely? Do customers stay informed? Are questions answered sufficiently and in a timely manner?

6. *Customer feedback.* How does your department know what customers are saying or thinking? What are the indicators in place to ensure that a standard is reached?

7. *Organization and supervision.* How efficient are procedures? How frequently do customers perceive they are monitored?

**Customer Service: Personal Dimension**

1. *Appearance.* A customer's reaction to service is strongly influenced by what one sees. Does appearance equate with professional?

2. *Attitude.* Body language and tone of voice. Like appearance, attitude is exposed for all to see. It is not always what is said but how it was delivered that makes all the difference.

3. *Attentiveness.* Being sensitive to customers and unique needs and expectations. Is care delivery really individualized? Do customers (patients, staff, and physicians) all feel that care provider is compassionate and interested in the customer?

4. *Tact.* Involves not only what message is sent but also the choice of words. Avoid offensive language. Avoid words that cause customer to become defensive (defensive reactions can cause immediate break in communication).

5. *Guidance.* Coaching, counseling, and even cheerleading for the customer.

*Continued*

**BOX 4-7—cont'd**

6. *Selling skills.* Healthcare, as any business, has selling services as an integral part of the service delivery business. With every customer encounter, one must become skillful at selling the services and expertise of the business. Cultivating relationships with customers is an important part of selling skills.

7. *Gracious problem solving.* Handling customer complaints promptly, before situation escalates to a situation that requires damage containment.

Modified from Katz, J. M., & Green, E. (1997). *Managing quality: A guide to system-wide performance management in health care* (2nd ed.). St. Louis:

## Action Tips

### COPING WITH CUSTOMER COMPLAINTS

Customers in any organization are the people who are serviced by the organization. For healthcare settings, customers include the patient, physician, interdepartmental colleagues, and other stakeholders in the corporation.

1. Always apologize for anything that goes wrong. It is not that the other party is necessarily right. Everything goes more smoothly when this is the perception.

2. Listen without interruption, even if the other party is raising his or her voice.

3. Identify the specific complaint before giving a reply.

4. There are people who enjoy complaining about everything except the real problem. Direct conversation to uncover the underlying dynamics of the situation. Keep emotions in check. Exhibiting professionalism assists in de-escalating a potentially volatile situation.

*Continued*

# Action Tips—Cont'd

## COPING WITH CUSTOMER COMPLAINTS—Cont'd

5. Never give excuses. No one wants to hear them and probably will not believe them. Excuses usually make the customer angrier. Never blame others. This is perceived as shirking your responsibilities.

6. When action is required, ensure that it is done as soon as possible. Follow up with the customer regarding the solution progress. Do everything possible to ensure that the customer has a positive attitude when leaving the department.

7. The more that the customer can be involved with the solution, the greater the resolution and customer satisfaction. This may be complicated, or it may be simply offering the customer a choice between alternatives.

8. Take even minor complaints seriously and address them with as much dedication as you would a major escalation.

9. Make every effort to follow-up in writing with the customer (i.e., follow-up letter to reassure patient/customer of your commitment to quality).

10. Use multiple monitoring tools to measure customer satisfaction. (Clerical areas frequently do phone surveys 48 to 72 hours after discharge. The results are incorporated into the organizational performance improvement model.)

moment" or a "tragic moment." The hundreds of personal encounters healthcare providers have with customers every single day have the potential for being categorized either way.

## BIBLIOGRAPHY

American College of Healthcare Executives. (1998). *Tutorial: ACHE board of governors examination.* Chicago: Author.

Burns, L. R. (1998). *Healthcare for the millennium.* AONE: The Executive Challenge (March).

Clark, R. (1998). *Financial scene—Presentation.* AONE: The Executive Challenge (March).

Cleverly, W. O. (1992). *Essentials of healthcare finance.* Rockville, MD: Aspen Publishers.

Dowd, R. (1988). Participative decision making in strategic management of resources. In H. Rowland & B. Rowland. *Nursing administration manual.* Rockville, MD: Aspen Publishers.

Drucker, P. (1995). *Managing in a time of change.* New York: Truman Tally Books/Dutton.

Finkler, S. (1992). *Budgeting concepts for nurse managers.* Philadelphia: W. B. Saunders.

Grady, G. (1995). *Developing and implementing outcomes-driven clinical pathways.* Houston: Saint Luke's Episcopal Hospital/Nashville: Business Networks.

Juhn, P. I. (1996). *The art and science of outcomes assessment: The roles of data, information, and decisions.* Oakland, CA: Kaiser Foundation Health Plan.

Kirk, R. (1988a). *Healthcare staffing and budgeting: Practical management tools.* Rockville, MD: Aspen Publishers.

Kirk, R. (1988b). *Healthcare quality and productivity: Practical management tools.* Rockville, MD: Aspen Publishers.

Kukla, B., & Weeks, L. (1994). *The financial management of hospitals.* Chicago: Health Administration Press.

Larson, E., & Peters, D. (1995). Integrating cost analyses in quality assurance. In H. Rowland & B. Rowland. *Nursing administration manual.* Rockville, MD: Aspen Publishers.

Marelli, T. (1997). *The nurse manager's survival guide.* St. Louis: Mosby.

Marker, C. (1995). Total quality management and the Marker Umbrella Model for quality management. In H. Rowland & B. Rowland. *Nursing administration manual.* Rockville, MD: Aspen Publishers.

Nelson, M. (1995). Budget in managing for productivity in nursing. In H. Rowland & B. Rowland. *Nursing administration manual.* Rockville, MD: Aspen Publishers.

Rowland, H., & Rowland, B. (1995a). *Nursing administration manual,* Vol. 1. Rockville, MD: Aspen Publishers.

Rowland, H., & Rowland, B. (1995b). *Nursing administration manual,* Vol. 2. Rockville, MD: Aspen Publishers.

Strasen, L. (1987). *Key business skills for nurse managers.* Philadelphia: J. B. Lippincott.

Wilson, C. (1995). Strategies for monitoring the cost-quality of care. In H. Rowland & B. Rowland. *Nursing administration manual.* Rockville, MD: Aspen Publishers.

# Chapter 5

# Networking

*A* *moment's insight is sometimes worth a life's experience.*
*Oliver Wendell Holmes*

*An eclectic definition, networking is a process of developing col-
lateral relationships or contacts that are utilized for information,
advice, and influence in obtaining personal and professional
goals, assistance in problem solving, moral support, and/or
socialization.*

Strasen (1987) reports that networking requires a con-
scious commitment of time, energy, and resources. She further asserts that the greatest benefit of networking is the
development of a broader base of both personal and professional power (*Action Tips* box). This process then
becomes a team effort rather than an individual or single
focus.

In order to sustain a firm commitment to networking,
Strasen (1987) offers the following advice:
- Routinely block out time on your calendar to make
  informal social telephone calls; contact colleagues to
  exchange information on such topics as open positions,
  problem-solving issues, and industry news.
- Return phone calls in a timely manner, and write thank-
  you notes for favors received.
- Take colleagues or potential network contacts out to
  lunch.

## Action Tips

*GOAL ATTAINMENT VIA NETWORKING*

1. Develop career goals. It is critical to develop a vision and subsequent long-term commitment (and confidence) to meet those goals.
2. Identify specific networks and network contacts that would be beneficial to cultivate:
   • Create a list of existing professional contacts that interface with your own goal-directed area of practice.
   • Initiate new contacts in areas where goals warrant development.
3. Actively participate in professional organizations.

## STRATEGIES FOR SUCCESS

To develop a broader base of network linkages and increased access to information to accomplish your goals, the following strategies are helpful (modified from Strasen, 1987):

• Subscribe to business and motivational journals outside the nursing profession. Broaden your perspectives by using strategies for success that have been identified by others. It is imperative to learn concepts from the business disciplines.

• Formulate your reference list of all network contacts into a business-card file format. Use fax or e-mail retrieval. Make it a habit to ask professionals for their business cards. Cards are retrievable files, and you can write personal notes easily on the back of each card as needed.

• Investing in yourself and your future is paramount. In the era of managed care and differentiated practice/case management models, managers and administrators

**Networking**

must pursue the appropriate credentials and academic preparation to be successful and credible. Become involved in speaker bureaus.

- Stay current with healthcare/industry changes. Administrators and managers must stay marketable and valued as a network link for others.
- Develop a strong self-image and active-listening skills.
- Develop skillful communication techniques. It is essential to be able to communicate the knowledge and special talents that you possesses to others.
- Develop the ability to make formal presentations to groups of all sizes and professional backgrounds. It is important to visualize yourself as confident, enthusiastic, and knowledgeable.

## MAKING NETWORK CONTACTS

As with anything risky, it takes *practice* to build self-confidence and determination. People are impressed with individuals who possess confidence and charisma. Be attentive to your personal characteristics and body language. Practice developing characteristics that denote confidence:

- Assertive, confident gait and handshake
- Healthy, physically fit appearance; proper and upright posture
- Good eye contact

A common strategic initiative is to telephone a particular leader or colleague that you admire. Whether you have met the individual previously or not is not important, and an action like this usually elicits a positive response. It is just as effective to write a flattering letter that reflects astute perceptions about the individual who is admired. In addition, with advancing technology, there are many vehicles used for communication and sources of networking (i.e., the Internet, interactive multimedia satellite services, professional organization directories, and conferences).

**Management Spotlight**

*PRACTICE*

- True professionals never stop practicing. Don't just *do a job*—develop the team's true potential.
- Trials and tribulations . . . Learn . . . Make corrections . . . Try again!

From Pritchett, P. (1997). *The team member handbook for teamwork.* Dallas: Pritchett & Associates.

There are specific practice guidelines that can assist in the networking process. However, equally important are these actions to be avoided (Strasen, 1987):

- Never alienate a network contact. You never know when or where he or she will appear again.
- Never treat colleagues other than how you would like to be treated.
- Never betray the confidentiality of information.
- Do not engage in gossip in professional situations.
- Never eliminate contacts with opposing views.
- Never be afraid to ask for assistance. Successful people know that asking for help is not a weakness—it is smart.
- Never miss an opportunity to network.
- Never miss an opportunity to establish a mentoring relationship and/or mentor someone else.

## FOUNDATION RELATIONSHIPS

Success in networking is directly related to the ability to establish long-lasting relationships. As a nurse, you need to constantly sell principles to the patient. As a leader, you must present new ideas to colleagues and employees; in other words, sell those ideas to them. Owens (1996) asserts that there are four basic relationships:

1. *Inward relationship* is how you relate to yourself or who you think you are. Your ability to establish relationships in other areas of life depends on the ability to relate positively with yourself.
   a. *Self-confidence* creates confidence in someone else's mind. *You* must believe in you before *I* can believe in you.
   b. *Self-acceptance* occurs when you know who you are (both strengths and weaknesses) and focus on using your strengths to conquer your weaknesses.
   c. *Self-image* is a mental picture of your ability to perform—what you can and cannot do.
   d. *Self-esteem* is how much value you place on who you are.
2. *Upward relationship* is how you relate to those in authority over you and those for whom you work.
3. *Downward relationship* is the reverse of upward—how you relate to those you have responsibility for or over whom you have authority.
4. *Outward relationship* is how you relate to people on a peer level or socially.

From his research, Owen (1996) asserts that successful people have the ability to develop strong relationships in the preceding four areas.

## MENTORING RELATIONSHIPS—BECOMING A MENTOR

According to Hagenow and McCrea (1994), mentoring is described as a teacher/student relationship in which the essence of success in leadership is evaluated through transference of ideas, experiences, and successful behavioral patterns. They also offer the following helpful hints to create the dynamic process to become a mentor:

- Focus on asking the right questions, not giving answers.
- Be confident enough to expose weakness and points of vulnerability.

- Give individuals a comprehensive view of the leadership role—the good, the bad, and the opportunities for improvement.
- Share your values and translate them into actions.
- Affirm the individual within; it amplifies learning. When there is an intrinsic development of self, there is a self-awareness toward new ideas, changing paradigms, and new information to the role of the leader.

## SELECTING THE RIGHT MENTOR: INITIATING THE RELATIONSHIP

To develop a dynamic relationship of mentorship, a process should be formalized so that the practice of nursing administration/management within the framework of theory can be synthesized. The process described as follows can be similarly interfaced with that of networking:

1. Perform a self-assessment. Identify your individual needs, goals, and vision (professionally, as well as personally).
2. Do homework on leadership styles, organizations, and systems and the strengths and weakness of nurse leaders in your own environment.
3. As networking circles grow, select someone who appears to share your own values, insights, and philosophy. Select someone who you would want as a counselor, teacher, and advisor. According to O'Brien (1989), mentoring relationships are formed; they are not based on an apprenticeship or role model.
4. Schedule uninterrupted time for an interview. Make sure that both parties openly share a mutual valuing of the mentoring process and a willingness to develop the relationship.
5. Formulate ground rules so that there is mutual respect and valuing of differences and learning experiences.
6. Formulate mutual goals to be evaluated periodically so that the relationship does not lose the mentorship dynamics.

Networking

## BIBLIOGRAPHY

Hagenow, N., & McCrea, M. (1994). A mentoring relationship. *Nursing Management, 25*(12): 42–43.

*God's little instruction book II: More inspirational wisdom on how to live a happy and fulfilled life.* (1984). Tulsa, OK: Honor Books.

O'Brien, M. (1989). Mentoring. In S. Cardin & C. Ward, eds. *Personnel management in critical care nursing.* Baltimore: Williams & Wilkins.

Owens, O. (1996). *The psychology of relationship selling.* Hollywood, FL: Lifetime Books.

Strasen, L. (1987). *Key business skills for nurse managers.* Philadelphia: J. B. Lippincott.

# Chapter 6

# Marketing Skills

*It is something to be able to paint a picture, or to carve a statue, and to make a few objects beautiful. But it is far more glorious to carve and paint the atmosphere in which we work, to affect the quality of the day—this is of the highest arts.*

*Henry David Thoreau*

## PLANNING AND MARKETING

Planning is necessary for survival in the current healthcare environment. Continuous strategic planning in a constantly changing environment allows organizations to respond to rapid changes, as well as to long-term trends. Strategic adaptation by healthcare organization leaders has resulted in new forms of healthcare delivery, integrated delivery systems, and new partnerships—all designed to serve the market better and more efficiently.

The need for effective marketing is equally imperative in a highly competitive environment. The direction in which the healthcare field is going suggests a more demanding market. The consumerism movement has not bypassed healthcare consumers. Consumer demand for more healthcare information has been supported by some large employers and buyers. The result has been the development of quality reporting in healthcare organizations.

### Marketing Mission and Objectives

Although the majority of healthcare marketing efforts historically have attempted to increase the volume and usage of

**183**

hospitals, medical practices, and other healthcare providers, according to Wopler (1995), the future objectives of most healthcare providers will be directed toward minimizing volume or use and, as a result, cost. In a managed care environment success may no longer be defined by high occupancy rates and high volume of procedures but by keeping the cost of *covered lives* low.

Volume will continue to be an objective for healthcare marketers. Managed care organizations will continue to look to increase the size of their memberships. Hospitals will, after downsizing if necessary, aim to maintain high occupancy level to cover their fixed costs (Wopler, 1995).

Strategic marketing is playing an increasingly important role in the effective management of health service organizations. Taylor (1994) suggest four reasons for the rise of strategic marketing in the healthcare industry:

1. A maturing in the area of traditional hospital planning, from an emphasis on physical plant and facilities to planning as a means to compete in dynamic competitive markets.
2. A greater understanding by hospitals that marketing is more than advertising.
3. A maturing of the hospital industry itself with consequent saturation.
4. A growth in hospital marketers' knowledge of the practical implementation of the strategic planning process.

Taylor further states that healthcare organizations will increasingly rely on positioning as a key marketing strategy to gain a sustainable competitive advantage. In addition, the provision of service quality and satisfaction are critical objectives in the strategic planning processes of healthcare organizations.

Marketing is a central activity of modern organizations. To survive and succeed, organizations must know their markets, attract sufficient resources, convert these resources into appropriate services, and communicate them to various consuming publics. In the hospital industry a marketing orientation is currently recognized as a necessary management function in a highly competitive and resource-constrained environment (Loubeau & Jantzen, 1998).

Hospitals can adopt one of four management orientations: *production* orientation, *product* orientation, *sales* orientation, or *marketing* orientation. Each orientation differs significantly in its approach and its likely market effects. Loubeau and Jantzen (1998) state that some publications refer to market orientation as being superior to the other three orientation approaches.

### Production orientation

Some hospitals focus on running a smooth operational process, even if customer needs must be bent to meet the requirements of that process. Loubeau and Jantzen (1998) described an example of this concept in place at a New York City hospital. The philosophy of this hospital suggested an attitude that the only way envisioned to improve profits was to reduce marketing and production costs. Outpatients are given only two appointment times; therefore large numbers of patients must wait long hours to see physicians, but the physicians are able to maximize their own efficiency in seeing patients.

### Product orientation

Some have argued that many organizations do not serve their markets adequately because their management is product oriented (Loubeau & Jantzen, 1998). Many organizations are strongly committed to their product and its value, even if the customers are having second thoughts or have an aversion to the process. The philosophy in this type of orientation suggests the attitude that the providers know what is best for the customer. Many services, such as oncology, obstetrics, and cardiology, model processes after other successful models.

Because a large amount of time, money, and other resources are invested in implementing these product lines, it is easy to overlook the fact that the model may not be meeting the specific community/customer needs or desires. Frequently cited as an example is the labor/delivery room/postpartum (LDRP) concept in obstetrical areas. Some hospitals continue to promote LDRP even though it is known that large percentages of women served by these hospitals have an aversion to this practice. According to Loubeau and Jantzen, product orientation leads to marketing myopia. If care is not taken, the industry or services decline rather than improve. These authors further assert that in product orientation communicating meanfully to users and packaging services to meet customer needs is not necessary.

### Sales orientation
Some organizations believe that they can substantially increase their market share through promotional efforts only. Rather than change the product or the service to make it more customer-oriented, these organizations invest in advertising or other forms of promotion.

### Marketing orientation
The significant difference in marketing orientation is that with this approach the organization assesses the needs of its customers (target markets) and satisfies them by design, communication, service delivery, and cost. This design is the one that hospitals should be attempting to achieve.

An adoption of a marketing orientation requires the following (Loubeau & Jantzen, 1998):

1. Management acknowledgment of the primacy of customer needs and desires in shaping the organization's strategic plan and operations; uses market research to obtain this information
2. Development of a new service mix appropriate to the target market and elimination of services that no longer meet the defined needs
3. Development of promotional activities to communicate with the target market
4. Development of an appropriate pricing strategy that is competitive, acceptable, and affordable
5. Development of efficient and innovative distribution strategies

Marketing in a healthcare organization can be perceived as a narrow scope of promotion, advertising, and public relations. However, this marketing concept centers on the need for the organization to be structured internally in such a way that the organization is responsive to changing customer needs. Key constituents or customers that marketing addresses include patients, physicians, and managed care organizations. By maintenance of a level of customer service and management support of marketing to ensure continued patient satisfaction for new and repeat business, the organization's marketing efforts are geared toward maximizing profits and an adequate return on investment.

Loubeau and Jantzen's study was the first national cross-sectional study of hospital marketing orientation in a managed care environment. The data revealed that in varying degrees hospitals are making strides in adopting a marketing orientation. However, only 30% of hospitals surveyed were highly marketing oriented. Major purchasers of healthcare have been asking for more information about the services their benefit dollars buy. In addition, as excess costs are eliminated from the hospital industry, hospitals may again turn to marketing orientation to retain managed care business by maintaining high levels of patient satisfaction.

## Issues Management as a Strategic Tool

Issues management is a systematic process for influencing the environment. An *issue* is a point of conflict between an organization and one or more of its publics (Reeves, 1993). Reeves describes four types of issues:

1. *Universal issues* have serious and imminent effects on a large number of people. Government action is expected since the issue is beyond the scope that can be handled by a private organization. (EXAMPLE: the energy crisis).

2. *Advocacy issues* are potential problems for most of the population that are identified by groups claiming to represent the broad public interest. Once again, the broad scope of the problem suggests that government intervention is appropriate. (EXAMPLE: health insurance reform).

3. *Selective issues* affect special interest groups. The costs of dealing with these issues, however, is generally passed on to the general population. (EXAMPLE: Medicaid reimbursement that results in cost shifting).

4. *Technical issues* are of little direct interest to the general public and are left to the experts. (EXAMPLE: hazardous waste disposal).

Currently issues management is recognized as a managerial responsibility involving identification of potential issues that may affect the organization and the mobilization of the organization's resources to strategically influence the course of those issues. Issues management and strategic planning should complement each other. The functions of issues management include (Reeves, 1993):

- Integrating public policy issues analysis into corporate strategic planning
- Monitoring standards of organizational performance to discover the opinions and values of key publics that may affect the organization's operations
- Developing and implementing codes of social accountability
- Assisting senior managers in making decisions about goals and operations that will influence or be influenced by public opinion
- Identifying, analyzing, and prioritizing the issues of greatest importance to the organization
- Creating practice plans for strategic responses to significant issues
- Carrying out the external communications part of the response plan
- Evaluating the effectiveness of the organization's issues and management program

With regard to purposes, the aim of strategic management is to make the organization more valuable for the stakeholders. The goal of issues management is to develop company policy and supporting action programs to participate in the public policy process of the resolution of sociopolitical and economic problems that will affect the organization's future visibility and well-being.

Taylor (1994) further describes four stakeholder groups: mixed-blessing, supportive, marginal, and nonsupportive. Taylor advises placing stakeholders in each of these categories and developing strategies for each group. For example, encourage involvement of supportive stakeholders. For nonsupportive stakeholders, you may need to use competitive marketing tactics for defense.

Strategic marketing is playing an increasingly important role in the effective management of health service organizations. Taylor (1994) cites four reasons for the recent rise of strategic marketing in the healthcare industry: (1) maturing in the area of traditional hospital planning as a means of competing in a dynamic competitive market; (2) greater understanding by hospitals that marketing involves more than advertising; (3) maturing of the hospital industry; and (4) growth in hospital marketers' knowledge of the practical implementation of the strategic planning process. Taylor further asserts that positioning is the key marketing strategy for gaining a sustainable competitive edge.

Marketing is a necessary business tool that encompasses all the operational components that satisfy customer needs. For the healthcare disciplines marketing becomes challenging and dynamic. Peter Drucker (1973) has described marketing as an integrated function of the entire business as viewed from the customer's point of view.

Marketing strives to accomplish various goals, for example (Strasen, 1987):

1. To maximize the marketplace's consumption of an organization's services or products
2. To maximize consumer satisfaction
3. To contribute to the quality of life of an individual or society

### The Four Ps of Marketing

McCarthy's simplified marketing classification system is referred to as the four Ps of marketing (Table 6-1 and Box 6-1):

- Product
- Promotion
- Price
- Place

**Table 6-1** Example Variables for Each of the Four Ps

|  | Business | Healthcare |
|---|---|---|
| Product | Quality | Professional competence |
|  | Styles | Expertise |
|  | Various options | Communication ability |
|  | Brand names | Problem solving, decision-making capabilities |
|  | Size | |
|  | Packaging | Teaching/management ability |
|  | | Resources developed through research, advanced education, experience |
| Promotion | Advertising | Business cards |
|  | Sales promotions | Resumés |
|  | Publicity | Professional attire/appearance |
|  | | Attitude |
|  | | Publications/presentations |
| Price | List price | Competitive pricing/costs |
|  | Discounts | Focus on resource consumption and cost rather than charges |
|  | Allowances | |
|  | Payment plans | |
|  | Credit terms | |
| Place | Channels of distribution | Professional organizations/journals |
|  | Coverage | Professional networking |
|  | Methods of distribution and transportation | Mentorships |
|  | | Community service |
|  | Inventory | Executive search firms |

Modified from Strasen, L. (1987). Key business skills for nurse managers. Philadelphia: J. B. Lippincott.

### *Product*

A *product* can be an object, service, activity, place, or idea that is capable of satisfying a customer desire. A *product line* is a group of similar services composed together to manage the cost, efficiency, effectiveness, and quality of the services.

---

**BOX 6-1**

## THE FOUR PS IN THE CLINICAL SETTING

**Sample Marketing Mix for "Same-Day" Surgery Program**

*Price*

      List price = $500 for minor procedures

    Discounts = Medicare deductible waived on weekends

                    5% discount for senior citizens

  Credit terms = 5% discount for cash

*Promotion*

Advertising = Sent out 100,000 direct-mail pieces

  Publicity = Local newspaper wrote full-page story on new

             "same-day" surgery program

*Place*

      Location = Free-standing "same-day" surgery building

             with free parking

Transportation = Free pick-up and delivery available

    Channels = Can be referred by private physician, as well

             as have minor surgery as a "walk-in"

*Product*

    Quality = Competent staff and physicians, but no-frills

          building to keep costs reasonable

Packaging = Billed as fast, safe, convenient alternative to in-

          patient surgery

  Options = All minor procedures available under general or

         local anesthesia

  Features = Convenient, reasonable healthcare service

---

From Strasen, L. (1987). *Key business skills for nurse managers.* Philadelphia: J. B. Lippincott.

---

Management of patient care by product line or by diagnosis requires cooperation and collaboration with the medical staff. The use of a critical pathway is an example of an attempt to capture product line management. The advantages of product line analysis are many; for example it:

- Provides better control and review of total resources
- Attaches all costs to the specific service and gives profit/loss information for a line of service

- Promotes detailed planning and interdepartmental teamwork
- Promotes optional efficiency and subsequent decision making

The Boston Consulting Group developed a product classification system to identify appropriate marketing strategies. It is based on the product's potential growth and profitability (Strasen, 1987). Fig. 6-1 shows the product classification matrix.

- *Cash cows* are products with low growth potential that are highly profitable. MARKETING STRATEGY: Maintain them, but use the profits to offset the losses from other ventures.
- *Rising stars* are products with high growth potential that are profitable. MARKETING STRATEGY: Increase promotional efforts to increase volume before product becomes a cash cow.
- *Question marks* are products with high growth potential that are not currently profitable. MARKETING STRATEGY: Specific efforts targeted toward specific need; however, effort must be directed to increase volume (in relationship to capacity).
- *Dogs* are products with low growth and low profitability potential. MARKETING STRATEGY: Attempt to divest service if it is a drain on organizational resources and cannot be financially offset by another service. Many organizations are outsourcing or contracting services to continue providing a service or product more cost-effectively.

### Promotion

The goal of promotion is to communicate, educate, and motivate the consumer to purchase of the product or service.

Marketing tools for promotion are categorized under advertising, personal selling, sales promotion, and publicity. The development and utilization of promotional tools specif-

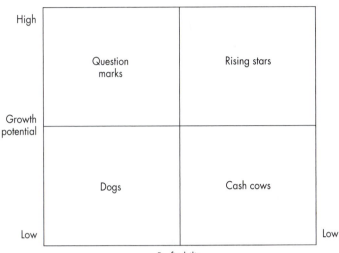

High

Growth
potential

Low

| Question marks | Rising stars |
| Dogs | Cash cows |

Low

Profitability

**Fig. 6-1**   The Boston Consulting Group's Product Matrix.
(From Strasen, L. [1987]. *Key business skills for nurse managers.*
Philadelphia: Lippencott.)

ically depend on the management decisions related to cost.
Allocation of resources depends on the goals and objectives
of the promotional campaign, the amount of resources and
promotional budget available, the market's perception of the
product, and the product life-cycle stage.

### Price
Pricing is the component of marketing that generates revenue
for the facility (Tables 6-2 and 6-3). Pricing objectives are
goals for specific profits, revenues, and market share for a
product (Strasen, 1987).

### Place (or distribution)
Distribution of products includes the following processes and
functions that take place from product development to product consumption: channels of distribution, locations of distribution, inventory, and transportation of products.

Marketing Skills

**Table 6-2**  Major Pricing Goals

| Pricing Goals/Objectives | Explanation |
|---|---|
| 1. Profit-maximizing pricing | Strives to determine the maximum price that the demand for a product will bear. |
| 2. Market-share pricing | Strives to identify the price that maximizes a company's share of the market. Short-term profits are sacrificed for long-term market domination. Profits are believed to follow the market domination. |
| 3. Market-skimming pricing | Includes a high price with a high profit, based on the assumption that the product is in high demand or has no competition. |
| 4. Promotional, loss-leader, and prestige pricing | Sets the price significantly higher or lower than the cost of the product to accomplish its purpose. Loss-leader pricing is setting the price lower than the cost or the competition to introduce the consumer to the company's products. The company makes up its losses when the consumer purchases other products. An example is a one-cent sale. Prestige pricing is setting unusually high prices to convey the image of a quality product through the pricing function. |
| 5. Target-profit pricing | To attain a satisfactory profit. |
| 6. Current-revenue pricing | To maximize current revenue for the company. |

From Strasen, L. (1987). *Key business skills for nurse managers.* Philadelphia: J. B. Lippincott.

## DEVELOPING A MARKETING PLAN

A marketing plan is a formal written proposal that details the organization's current position, projected goals and objectives for profits and gaining market share, and strategies to obtain and evaluate the goals (*Action Tips* box). The following are the main elements of a marketing plan (Strasen, 1987):

**Table 6-3**  Pricing Factors and Methods

| Pricing Factor | Pricing Method | Definition |
|---|---|---|
| Cost of product | 1. Mark-up pricing | Determined by multiplying cost by a certain percentage. |
| | 2. Cost-plus pricing | Determined by adding a fixed amount to the cost. |
| | 3. Target pricing | Price is the one that yields a specific profit above the total costs at a particular demand level. |
| Demand for product | 1. Perceived-value pricing | The price is based on the consumer's perceptions of the value of the product. |
| | 2. Price-discrimina-tion pricing | The price of a product varies from one consumer to another, one time to another, and one place to another, based on the perceptions of value. Example: seasonal hotel rates. |
| Competition | 1. Going-rate pricing | Determined by the collective wisdom of the marketplace; is the price the market will bear. |
| | 2. Sealed-bid pricing | This pricing is the lowest price a company is willing to be paid for a product, given that other competitors are vying for the contract. |

From Strasen, L. (1987). *Key business skills for nurse managers.* Philadelphia: J. B. Lippincott.

1. *Situational analysis.* An organization/department/service area must assess the external environment (marketplace) and the internal strengths and weaknesses to position itself to determine a strategic vision and set future goals/objectives. There are several analytical methods to implement an assessment.
2. *Marketing goals/objectives.* These identify broad marketing goals and the subsequent objectives that are measurable and obtainable to meet the identified goals.

# Action Tips

3. *Marketing strategy.* This methodology is used to achieve predetermined goals and objectives. It involves marketing mix (the combination of the four Ps), marketing expenditure (percentage of budget allocated), and market allocation (amount of resources committed to marketing project).

4. *Marketing action plan.* This formal component includes written action steps, responsibilities and accountability, and time frame involved.

5. *Continual evaluation and revision.* This process is the control function for the plan. Goals and objectives are continually revised as the healthcare market and the external environment rapidly changes.

Two characteristics that are critical to optimum success of any organization are foresight and customer-focused service delivery. Many authors agree that responding to the customer's needs is the ultimate goal of marketing. Through the turbulence of healthcare changes, nursing interfaces interdepartmentally with many ancillary-support departments and services. Nursing service is greatly challenged to increase the market's perception of the value of its goods and services. In other words, the needs of all services, employees, and other contributors to healthcare delivery must be evaluated and prioritized secondary to the customer (however, *customer* is defined in the particular conceptual framework of the organization).

The previous matrix can be juxtaposed differently depending on the frame of reference and strategic approach taken:

*Positive* (strengths/opportunities) and *negative* (weaknesses/threats)

*Present* (strengths/weaknesses) and *future* (threats/opportunities)

Forces and trends are usually divided into these categories: political, economic, social, and technological.

### Snow Card Technique

A simple yet effective group process for developing SWOT lists (Fig. 6-2) combines brainstorming with grouping data into categories. Each of the individual answers is written on a 3 × 5 card. The cards are taped to the wall according to common themes.

As with any approach, data are discussed, compared, and contrasted to determine the strategic issues/goals and the prioritization of actions to prepare for effective strategies.

SWOT Analysis (Example)    Remarkably Productive Questions:
1. What major external opportunities are present?
2. What major external threats are faced in organization?
3. What are the major internal strengths?
4. What are the major external weaknesses?

**Internal**

**Strengths**                                                      **Weaknesses**

Staff expertise/competencies
Financial position/productivity
Hospital leadership dynamics
Physical plant and logistics
Quality of services and programs
MD partnerships

**Opportunities**                                                   **Threats**

Marketplace
Location/Transportation

Referral patterns                          Competition
Improved technology                        Changing population
Expanded services                            and demographics
Legislative changes                        Decreasing reimbursement
Expanded contract capability               Loss of FP physicians

**External**

**Fig. 6-2**   Popular Environmental and Situational Assessments.
*SWOT:* Strengths/Weaknesses/Opportunities/Threats.

## Strategic Planning

Amidst turbulent healthcare changes and managed care re-engineering efforts, a critical component of organizational leadership is strategic planning. Strategic planning is best described as a disciplined effort to create a comprehensive vision. In the process strategic planning produces fundamental decisions and actions that shape, guide, and give purpose to an organizational entity. Strategic planning is one way to help organizations and communities deal with changing circumstances. Specifically, *strategic planning:*

- Focuses on performance improvement but relies on identification and resolution of issues
- Emphasizes assessment of the environment (inside and outside the organization)
- Is action oriented and embraces qualitative shifts in direction and includes a broad range of contingency plans
- Is guided by a vision of success

Many authors agree that strategic planning can benefit an organization in many ways, for example, to:

- Think strategically and develop effective and result-oriented strategies
- Clarify future endeavors and direction
- Make current decisions in the light of future consequences
- Develop a defensible and comprehensive basis for decision making
- Exercise maximum direction in the areas under organizational control
- Make decisions interdepartmentally
- Solve organization problems and improve performance
- Become highly effective in a rapidly changing world
- Build teamwork expertise

Even though strategic planning can provide all the above benefits, not all approaches are equal and useful since a number of variables govern the successful use of each approach.

### Corporate approaches to strategic planning

This discussion focuses on six models of or approaches to planning. The strategic planning process includes general policy direction, direction setting, situational assessment, strategic issues and identification, strategy development, decision making, and action and evaluation (Bryson, 1988).

**Harvard policy model.** The Harvard Policy Model (HPM) is the most widely cited model of public and non–profit-sector strategic planning (Bryson, 1988). The main purpose of the HPM is to help an organization develop the best fit between itself and the environment—to craft the best strategy for the organization. The systematic assessment of strengths, weaknesses, opportunities, and threats (SWOT analysis) is the primary strength of the Harvard model. Its weakness is that it does not offer specific advice on how to develop strategies except to note that effective strategies will build on strengths, take advantage of opportunities, and overcome or minimize weaknesses and threats.

**Strategic planning systems.** This approach is viewed as a system in which managers make, implement, and control decisions across functions and levels in the organization. It is built on mission, strategies, budgets, and controls. The strength of these systems is the attempt to coordinate the various elements of the organization's strategy across levels and functions. Their weakness is that excessive comprehensiveness, prescription, and control tend to drive out attention to the mission, strategy, and organizational structure (Bryson, Van de Ven, & Roering, 1987).

**Stakeholder management approaches.** A stakeholder is any group or individual who is affected by or can affect the future of the organization. Corporate strategy is usually effective only if it satisfies the needs of multiple groups; therefore many argue that an organization's mission and values should be formulated in stakeholder terms. The strengths of the stakeholder model are its recognition of the complementary and competing claims placed on the organization to satisfy at least the key stakeholders to survive. Its weakness is the absence of criteria with which to judge competition effectively and the need for advice on how to develop strategies to deal with various interest groups.

**Portfolio models.** This approach views a corporation as a portfolio of businesses with diverse potentials that can be balanced to manage return and cash flow. An example of the portfolio model is the Boston Consultant Group (BCG) model in which a relationship is postulated among unit costs, potential profit, and volume. The strength of portfolio approaches is that they provide a method of measuring certain entities (e.g., services, investment options, proposals, problems) against dimensions of strategic importance (e.g., share growth, position, attractiveness). The weaknesses include the difficulty of knowing what the appropriate dimensions are and the problems associated with classifying entities against the dimensions.

**Competitive analysis.** Competitive analysis assumes that by analyzing the forces that shape an industry one can predict the general level of profit and success of a particular strategy for a strategic business unit (SBU). The strength of this method is that it provides a way of assessing industries facing SBUs. The weakness is that it is difficult to isolate an industry and what forces affect it; the key to success is often collaboration, not competition.

**Strategic issue management.** This approach is a process that focuses attention on recognition and resolution of an issue. Its strength is that it affords the ability to quickly recognize and analyze key issues. Its weakness is that it offers no specific advice on exactly how to frame the issues.

*STRATEGIC NEGOTIATIONS.* This approach applies to organizations in which negotiation is increasingly becoming a way of life for leaders and managers. An example is the collaboration of federal, state, and local agencies in several locations to develop a coordinated investment strategy designed to meet the objectives of each agency. The strength of this approach is the recognition that power is something to be shared. The weakness is that although it can aid in reaching politically accepted results, it may not be helpful in ensuring the technical workability or responsibility of the results.

*LOGICAL INCREMENTALISM.* This strategy is a loosely linked group of decisions handled incrementally. Its strength is the ability to handle complexity and change; in addition, it emphasizes minor decisions and can be informal. Its weakness is that there is no guarantee that the incremental strategies will add up to the fulfillment of corporate purposes.

### An effective strategic planning approach

Bryson (1988) suggests that whatever the strategic approach taken, it needs to be orderly, deliberate, participative, and strategically planned so that it will yield actions, results, and evaluation methods. The general steps for most strategic plans include the following:

1. Initiating and agreeing on a strategic planning process. Negotiate agreement with key internal (or external) decision makers and delineate which persons are to be involved. This step includes:
   - Purpose of effort
   - Steps in preferred process
   - Form and timing of reports
   - Group membership (role and function), responsibility, and accountability
2. Clarifying the organizational mandates: relevant ordinances, constraints, legislation, and contracts with which the organization must comply.
3. Clarifying the organizational mission and values:
   - Know the social justification for its existence
   - Develop a mission statement (from stakeholder's analysis)
4. Assessing the external environment. Opportunities and threats can be discovered by monitoring a variety of political, economic, social, and technological forces and trends (PEST). PEST is an appropriate acronym because organizations usually must respond by reengineering, and change can be quite painful.
5. Assessing the internal environment. To identify its internal strengths and weaknesses, the organization could monitor resources, current strategies, and performance improvement data. The relative lack of performance criteria and information causes major organizational conflicts. It is difficult to evaluate the relative effectiveness of alternative strategies, resource allocation, organizational designs, and distribution of power.
6. Identifying the strategic issues facing an organization. Strategic issues include the fundamental policy questions affecting the organizational mandates, philosophy, mission, core values, services, stakeholders, fiscal status, and management.

7. Formulating strategies to manage the issues:
   - Identify practical alternatives and visions of success
   - Identify barriers to achieving those successes
   - Develop (through team) major proposals for achieving alternatives and successes
   - Develop actions needed and time lines
   - Detail work program:
     —Technically workable
     —Politically acceptable (relatively) to key stakeholders
     —Congruent with organizational mission/core values
8. Formalizing an effective organizational vision. Articulating a vision of success can come as early in the strategic planning process as needed; it acts as a stabilizing force in the process. This written statement includes a short and inspiring description of the rest of the organization:
   - Mission
   - Basic strategies
   - Performance criteria
   - Decision roles and ethical standards expected of employees

The planning vision should motivate people and be challenging enough to spur them into action. Tables 6-4 and Fig. 6-3 depict a typical strategic plan process flow chart. Fig. 6-4 shows a sample strategic planning worksheet.

In a strategic approach to planning the process begins with an in-depth assessment of the organization, its mission, and its environment. There should be an attitude of openness to challenge traditional methods, conventional wisdom, and existing paradigms. Strategic thinking enables a manager to consider how to change the environment rather than simply reacting to it. Changing the paradigm takes time, effort, resources, creativity, and risk taking.

### Conducting the external assessment

A critical component to any strategic approach is a detailed assessment of both the external and internal environments. Assessing the external environment in today's turbulent

**Table 6-4** The Strategic Planning Process

| Planning Steps | Time Frame | Responsible Person |
|---|---|---|
| 1. Develop a planning procedure and gain agreement from key individuals | Two meetings held within 2 weeks | Administrator, planning director, and planning consultant |
| 2. Assess organization mission statement | Two-day retreat | Administrator, board chair, and physician representative |
| 3. Assess external environment | Six weeks | Planning director, planning consultant, and planning staff |
| 4. Assess internal environment | Six weeks (simultaneously with external environment) | Planning director, planning consultant, and planning staff |
| 5. Develop organizational goals | Two weeks following circulation of internal and external assessment data | Administrator, board planning committee, planning director, consultant, and staff |
| 6. Formulate strategic options for accomplishing each goal | One month after agreement on organizational goals | Administrator, planning director, consultant, board planning committee, and staff planning teams |
| 7. Select and develop strategic options to be implemented | One week after formulation of strategic options | Administrator, planning director, planning consultant, board planning committee, and staff planning teams |
| 8. Approve the strategic plan with specific options, costs, and estimated | First board meeting following final selection of strategic options | Governing body |

**Table 6-4**    The Strategic Planning Process—Con't

| Planning Steps | Time Frame | Responsible Person |
|---|---|---|
| implementation dates supplied by the governing body | | |
| 9. Develop action plan and implementation schedule for each chosen strategic option | Varies with the complexity of each option; however, no longer than 1 month will be allowed for any option | Administrator, planning director, and various department heads |

From Wopler, L. (1995). *Health care administration.* Rockville, MD: Aspen Publishers.

milieau takes meticulous attention to detail and an ability to assimilate a large quantity of data with significant but unavoidable gaps (Wopler, 1995). Wopler presents the following six objectives for this process:

1. Classify and order information flows generated by outside organizations
2. Identify and analyze current important issues that will affect the organization
3. Detect and analyze the weak signals of emerging issues that will affect the organization
4. Speculate on the likely future issues that will have a significant impact on the organization
5. Provide organized information for development of the origination's purpose, mission, objectives, internal assessment, and strategy
6. Foster strategic thinking throughout the organization

An external environmental assessment assists those involved in the strategic planning process to identify the potential threats and opportunities for the healthcare facility.

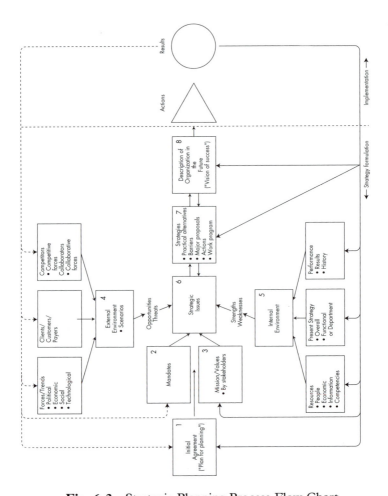

**Fig. 6-3** Strategic Planning Process Flow Chart.

(From Bryson, J. [1988]. *Strategic planning for public and nonprofit organizations.* San Francisco: Jossey-Bass.)

## Strategic Issue Identification

1. What is the issue? Be sure to phrase the issue as a question about which your organization can take some type of action.

2. Why is this an issue? What is it about the conjunction of mission and mandates, external opportunities and threats, or internal strengths and weaknesses that makes this an issue?

3. What are the consequences of not addressing this issue?

## Practical Alternatives or Visions

What are the practical alternatives, dreams, or visions we might want to pursue to address this strategic issue?

1. Practical alternative or vision # _____

2. Practical alternative or vision # _____

3. Practical alternative or vision # _____

## Barriers Identification

1. Barrier # _____

2. Barrier # _____

3. Barrier # _____

*Continued*

**Fig. 6-4, *A*** Sample Strategic Planning Worksheet.

(From Bryson, J. [1988]. *Strategic planning for public and nonprofit organizations.* San Francisco: Jossey-Bass.)

Marketing Skills

### Major Proposals

What are the major proposals we might pursue either to achieve the practical alternatives, or visions directly or to overcome the barriers to their realization?

Strategy # _____

Strategy # _____

Strategy # _____

### Major Actions

What major actions with existing staff and within existing job descriptions must be taken within the next year to implement the strategies or proposals? What is the financial impact for proposed strategies?

Major action # _____

Major action # _____

Major action # _____

### Action Steps

What action steps must be taken in the next six months to implement the proposals and who is responsible for the action step?

1. Action step # _____ Person responsible _____ Projected timeline_____

2. Action step # _____ Person responsible _____ Projected timeline_____

3. Action step # _____ Person responsible _____ Projected timeline_____

**Figure 6-4, *B*** Sample Strategic Planning Worksheet.

The external environment can be systematically assessed by using the following topics as a guide:

1. *Macroenvironment.* Includes major trends and events taking place outside the specific environment (i.e., industry trends, global economy, reimbursement changes).

2. *Regulatory environment.* Focuses on recent or expected changes that directly affect the organization.

3. *Economic environment.* Includes trends, events, and economic indicators specific to the marketplace in which the organization operates. In addition, it targets the assessment of areas and services of potential growth, the strength and impact of managed care, and the impact on service delivery.

4. *Social environment.* Includes issues such as the public health status of the marketplace, health impacts of generalized social behaviors (e.g., poor diet, sexually transmitted diseases, smoking, substance abuse), and demographic changes and trends in the marketplace.

5. *Political environment.* Addresses factors such as legislative activities and decisions at local, state, and federal levels.

6. *Competitive environment.* Attempts to define the strengths and weaknesses of other organizations that are seeking to offer similar services. Also includes any recent or expected changes in partnerships and strategic alliances in the marketplace.

7. *Technological environment.* Includes assessments of recent advances in pharmaceuticals, genetics, and high-technology equipment or procedures.

### Conducting the internal assessment

The internal assessment not only identifies organizational strengths and weaknesses, it also evaluates them in relation to the specific external opportunities and threats that have been identified. According to Wopler (1995), the organization can be divided into 10 operating components to facilitate this

## Management Spotlight

*BRING TALENT TO THE TEAM*

- Give your teammates good reasons to believe in you.
- Keep getting better at what you do.
- The team is only as strong as its weakest link.

From Pritchett, P. (1997). *The team member handbook for teamwork.* Dallas: Pritchett & Associates.

phase of the process. The 10 components evaluated in the internal assessment are:

1. *Management.* Includes evaluation of the number of levels, the strength of each level as a whole and the individuals in that level, management skills, and formal delegation of decision-making authority.
2. *Human resources.* Focuses on evaluation of the skill levels in technical areas, availability of appropriately prepared personnel, recruitment and retention track record, and efficiency in scheduling.
3. *Finance.* Includes evaluation of the availability and use of capital funds, use of operating revenues, ratio analyses, budget variances, and internal control mechanisms.
4. *Marketing.* Includes analysis of the characteristics of current patients, such as payor source, acuity, demographics, origin, and destination; referral sources; review of the current level of usage of services or product lines offered; mechanisms for service delivery; and success rate.
5. *Clinical systems.* Targets evaluation of output measures of volume and quality, level of technology needed, and skills and knowledge base of clinicians.
6. *Organization culture.* What effect culture has on the actual productivity of an organization is uncertain.

However, this assessment should assist in the organizational development of a value system and behavioral expectations that support the mission.

7. *Physical plant.* For planning purposes the primary interest is whether or not the plant serves to consolidate or facilitate future growth or change.

8. *Information systems.* According to Wopler (1995), this component typically has very high levels of dissatisfaction in healthcare provider organizations. This assessment should evaluate the system's ability to link the financial, clinical, and marketing information systems.

9. *Organization structure.* Includes analysis of the linkages between human resources, technologies, marketing, and management collaboration.

10. *Leadership abilities.* Highlights evaluation of the demonstrated leadership of the organization's senior and executive managers, governing body, and department heads. This is a particularly sensitive area to evaluate; thus, unfortunately, it is sometimes left out of the process.

In converting the internal and external data into meaningful information, it is important to compile a list of the organization's internal strengths and weaknesses and the opportunities and threats that exist in the external environment (SWOT analysis).

At the point in the process when it is time to select and develop strategies, Peter Drucker (Wopler, 1995) warns of the top four common mistakes that can be made:

- Failure to test the new strategy before full implementation.
- Failure to make the necessary changes because that is not the way it was conceived or proposed. This can cause a potentially successful strategy to fail.
- Failure to develop and propose radical strategies.
- Assumption that there is just one right strategy for each goal and that the role of the planning committee is to figure out which one it is.

Marketing Skills

## THE FIVE DEADLY BUSINESS SINS

Peter Drucker (1995) asserts that there are avoidable mistakes that will harm the best of businesses. He states that the common thread in each organizational downfall is at least one of the following deadly business sins:

1. *The worship of high profit margins and premium pricing.* This is easily the most common sin. Premium pricing always creates a market for the competitor. High profit margins do not equal maximum profits.

2. *Mispricing a new product by charging what the market will bear.* This approach also creates risk-free opportunity for the competition.

3. *Cost-driven pricing.* The only thing that works is price-driven costing. As soon as you put a profit margin on top of costs, when product hits the market, you are forced to start cutting prices or redesigning initiatives at enormous costs. Subsequently, you start culminating enormous losses and may even drop the product when it was only priced incorrectly. Cost-led pricing destroyed U.S. industries and caused foreign products to lead the world market because of their price-led costing strategy instead.

4. *Slaughtering tomorrow's opportunity on the altar of yesterday.* Holding onto traditional methods and service delivery can stifle opportunities that can change the future. Opportunities often have small windows and require risk taking.

5. *Feeding problems and starving opportunities.* All you can hope to gain from problem-solving is damage control; opportunities produce results and growth. Opportunities facing the business or organization are actually every bit as demanding and difficult as problems and should have even greater resources assigned to them.

Peters and Waterman (1984) developed eight interrelated criteria that characterize successfully managed "excellent" companies, and they are still valid today:

- A bias for action (identify problems and implement resolutions)

- Close to the customer (emphasize quality, reliability, and service)
- Autonomy for entrepreneurship (never suppress a good idea)
- Productivity through people (people are the most valuable resource)
- Hands on, value driven (people live the business; core values)
- Stick to the knitting (do not go at odds with core businesses)
- Simple form, lean staff
- Simultaneous loose-tight properties (exhibit core values and promote autonomy and decentralization)

## BIBLIOGRAPHY

Bryson, J. (1988). *Strategic planning for public and nonprofit organizations: A guide to strengthening and sustaining organizations.* San Francisco: Jossey-Bass.

Bryson, J., Van de Ven, A., & Roering, W. (1987). Strategic planning and the revitalization of the public service. In R. Denhardt & E. Jennings (Eds.). *Toward a new public service.* Columbia, MO: Extension Publications, University of Missouri.

Drucker, P. (1995). *Managing in a time of great change.* New York: Truman Talley Books/Dutton.

Drucker, P. (1973). *Tasks, responsibilities, and practices.* New York: Harper & Row.

Loubeau, P., & Jantzen, R. (1998). The effect of managed care on hospital marketing orientation. *Journal of Healthcare Management, (43),* 3, 229–241.

Peters, T., & Waterman, R. (1984). *In search of excellence: Lessons from America's best-run companies.* New York: Harper & Row.

Reeves, P. (1993). Issues management: The other side of strategic planning. *Hospital and Health Services Administration, 38*(2), 229–241.

Strasen, L. (1987). *Key business skills for nurse managers.* Philadelphia: J. B. Lippincott.

Taylor, S. (1994). Distinguishing service quality from patient satisfaction in developing healthcare strategies. *Hospital and Health Services Administration, 39*(2), 221–233.

Wopler, L. (1995). *Health care administration.* Rockville, MD: Aspen Publishers.

# Part Three
# Policy
# Responsibilities

# Chapter 7

# Politics for the Healthcare Manager

*I believe that every right implies a responsibility; every opportunity, an obligation; every possession, a duty.*
*John D. Rockefeller, Jr.*

*Politics* is a complex process whereby each team member interacts toward common goals and objectives within an organization. The complexity evolves from the underlying dynamics of the group because each team member has differing self-interests, viewpoints, priorities, and experiences.

## POLITICAL MYTHS AND REALITIES

There are fundamental concepts that are essential for any healthcare leader to acknowledge. These concepts should assist the leader in making a comprehensive assessment of situations and subsequent decision making.

1. Who are the stakeholders and team players?
   - What position or role does each play in the organization?
   - What are the strengths and weaknesses of each player?
   - What are the existing coalitions already established?
2. How much influence does each player have? What is the area of expertise in each player that the healthcare manager wants to access?
   - What is the manager's contribution to the rest of the stakeholders?
   - Who are the formal and informal leaders?

**217**

3. What are the projected outcomes of the interactions? How is success measured?

*Power is neutral, neither positive nor negative. It is the means by which goals are accomplished.*

*Powerlessness, in congruence with the previous definition of power, denotes the inability to accomplish goals.*

According to Strasen (1987), one should fear "powerless" people rather than powerful ones. Individuals without power are often compelled to resort to unhealthy and unethical methods to accomplish their goals, such as undermining, manipulation, dishonesty, and sabotaging efforts. Powerful people, on the other hand, are confident enough to be direct and "up front" in the words and actions they use to accomplish their goals.

Generally, it is suggested that there are five interpersonal bases of power: legitimate, reward, coercive, referent, and expert (Swansburg, 1990). Power is simply the capacity to ensure the outcomes that one wishes. The five interpersonal bases of power are:

- *Legitimate power* is a person's ability to influence because of the position he or she occupies. Legitimate power is dependent on subordinates.
- *Reward power* involves using rewards to gain the cooperation of subordinates. Followers may respond to directions or requests if the leader can provide valued rewards as incentives to perform better.
- *Coercive power* is the ability to persuade through the perception that there is no choice. Usually there is a negative aspect, such as punishment, related to coercion. Coercive power is used to correct nonproductive or destructive behavior. The risk is that this approach could have the opposite effect on employees; employees may "act out" under perceived duress (i.e., absenteeism, sabotage, hostility).
- *Referent power* is a power that is part of the personality of an individual. A charismatic, joyful leader can influence people because of his or her personality and style. Peo-

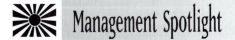

## Management Spotlight

### PLAY YOUR POSITION

- It's tough to achieve a coordinated team effort when people get sloppy and let things fall through the cracks.
- Set clear expectations, duties, or standards of performance.
- You support your colleagues best by playing your position to perfection.

From Pritchett, P. (1997). *The team member handbook for teamwork.* Dallas: Pritchett & Associates.

ple are usually drawn to this type of leader and enjoy being around them.

- *Expert power* is the ability to influence people based on a special knowledge base. The individual is highly valued as an expert in a particular area. An example is the clinical nurse specialist, who can easily change practice patterns based on the respect of his or her expertise.

People use power to accomplish goals and to strengthen their positions in the organization. The use of power is legitimate when it is used in an equitable and ethical way to achieve organizational, group, or individual objectives (Swansburg, 1990). A good manager desires power to influence the behavior of employees for the good of the organization, not for personal growth (Table 7-1).

## DEVELOPING POLITICAL SAVVY

It is imperative for an administrator or manager to be able to use the political process to accomplish service area goals effectively within a functional and viable healthcare organization (*Action Tips* box).

**Table 7-1** Myths and Realities of Power and Politics

| Myths | Realities |
| --- | --- |
| 1. Hard work and competence always result in success. | 1. Success is situational. The boss defines what hard work and competence are. |
| 2. Being fired means you are incompetent. | 2. There may be no relationship between competence and being fired; often it is a subjective perception of "fit." |
| 3. Performance appraisals can be objective if done properly. | 3. Performance appraisals are always subjective. |
| 4. Office politics is a nasty game, played by bad people. | 4. Office politics is a normal organization process. |
| 5. Individuals are either politically savvy, or they are not. | 5. Political savvy is learned. |
| 6. Top management possesses all the political clout. | 6. There are some people who are low on the organizational chart who are actually more powerful than some managers. |
| 7. It is possible to "rise above" the politics in an organization if you are a responsible, ethical manager. | 7. It is impossible not to be involved in politics of the organization if you are performing your job appropriately. |

From Strasen, L. (1987). *Key business skills for nurse managers.* Philadelphia: J. B. Lippincott.

## Action Tips

### DEVELOPING POLITICAL SAVVY

The following are strategies that managers should consider in developing political savvy.

- Use a careful interview and employee selection process to reduce potential conflict situations in the department.

*Continued*

## Action Tips–Cont'd

- Although diversity is healthy for organizational growth, it is important for administrators and managers to set the expectation for employee support. Approach problems directly and promptly to ensure employee support. Administrators and managers are not effective and are perceived as dishonest when they avoid dealing with a problem.
- Consistently work on developing cooperative and supportive relationships with colleagues for long-term success. Dysfunctional management groups are typical when cooperation is not present and peers compete with, "squeal" on, and undermine one another.
- When you are considering a new position, the most important factor in that decision is your relationship with the new superior. It is critical to select a political arena in which you can survive and be successful.
- Cheerfulness and kind words are excellent weapons against defeat.
- Identify the credible grapevine and informal leaders. Pass on "honest" information that is important to be circulated quickly. The grapevine can also be used to test the organizational climate at a specific point in time.
- A manager or administrator should learn to read what the superiors read. By reading what the boss reads, you have an insight into what the boss is thinking and believes is important.
- Actively listen to secretaries. They have access to privileged information, conversations, and intuitive feelings. They can be advocates and protectors of leaders in the political underground of an organization. A good secretary can keep the manager on top of issues on a continual basis.
- Make the decision that learning to "fit" into an organizational culture and learning the rules of the game to obtain goals is often more important than being right. In other

*Continued*

## Action Tips–Cont'd

words, pick battles carefully while attempting to change the present culture. Under no circumstances, however, should integrity, personal values, and moral fortitude be compromised.

- Use negotiation strategies, rather than compromise, as a cooperative effort, whereby participants are persuaded to strive for mutually valued goals. One mechanism is to rephrase individual goals so that one is assisting others in obtaining their goals as a strategy to obtain one's individual goal.
- Identify and align yourself with powerful people in the organization.
- Work diligently; volunteer for extra projects and responsibilities.
- Know the job, the organization, the business, and the healthcare industry.
- Know the competition, market targets, and assessments.
- Stay visible and highly assertive.
- Develop excellent communication skills.
- Know the preferences and vision of superiors.
- View all problems as opportunities to create something better.

Modified from Strasen, L. (1987). Key business skills for nurse managers. Philadelphia: Lippencott.

Cavanaugh (1985) published five possible strategies to deal with the politics of a healthcare organization. She defines the term associated with each category as a strategy used by the manager. Cavanaugh coined the term *gamesmanship* as the process by which the strategies are used.

1. *Disengagement* is a proactive refusal to defend oneself on another's terms. The manager purposely chooses not to pursue the issue further at a particular time.
2. *Offense* means taking charge and making the commitment to pursue a particular goal at all costs. The man-

ager chooses to champion the initiative until the end. This approach requires tenacity and perserverence.

3. *Defense* is the strategy used in response to an advance by another party into an individual's territory.

4. *Building a coalition* means teaming up in a collaborative effort to achieve mutual goals.

5. *Exploiting* an opportunity is simply using a situation to one's own advantage. This does not necessarily mean that an individual takes advantage of another; instead, the person seizes an opportunity to move forward. Highly effective leaders use this strategy, which involves proactive and keen insight, strategic vision, sense of timing, flexibility, and adaptability, as a leadership attribute.

## HEALTHCARE POLICY

Over many decades the role of government in the organization, financing, and delivery of healthcare services in the United States has evolved from that of a highly controlled provider and protector of public health to that of a major financial underwriter of an enormous and essentially private enterprise.

The vast majority of healthcare expenditure by the federal government is managed by the Department of Health and Human Services (DHHS). The major subdivisions of the DHHS include the Public Health Service (PHS), the Health Care Financing Administration (HCFA), the Social Security Administration (SSA), the Administration for Children and Families, and the Administration on Aging. It may be difficult to remember which services are provided by DHHS. Therefore Fig. 7-1 presents an organizational map that provides an overview of where agencies fall on the organizational grid.

### Public Health Service

The Public Health Service (PHS) continues to broaden the scope of its activities. The broad mission of this organization is to promote protection and advancement of the nation's physical and mental health.

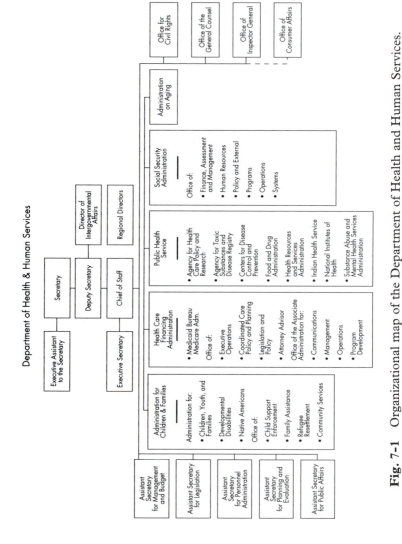

**Fig. 7-1**   Organizational map of the Department of Health and Human Services.

(From Calkins, D., Fernandopulle, R., & Marino, B. [1995]. *Health care policy*. Cambridge, MA: Blackwell Science.)

- The *Agency for Health Care Policy and Research* (AHCPR) was established by the Omnibus Budget Reconciliation Act of 1989. This federal agency is charged with producing and disseminating relevant scientific and policy information about the quality, medical effectiveness, and cost of healthcare.
- The *Agency for Toxic Substances and Disease Registry* (ATSDR) was established as an operating agency within the PHS by the Secretary of Health and Human Services in 1983. The mission of this agency is to carry out the health-related responsibilities of the Comprehensive Environmental Response, Compensation and Liability Act of 1980.
- The *Centers for Disease Control and Prevention* (CDC), established as an agency within the PHS by the Secretary of Health, Education and Welfare in 1973, is charged with protecting the public health of the nation by providing leadership and direction in the prevention and control of diseases and other preventable conditions. In addition, this agency is charged with responding to public health emergencies.
- The *Food and Drug Administration* (FDA), which was created through the Agriculture Appropriations Act of 1931, is charged with protecting the health of the nation against impure and unsafe foods, drugs, cosmetics, and other potential hazards.
- The *Health Resources and Services Administration* (HRSA) has leadership responsibility in the PHS for general health services and resource issues relating to access, equity, quality, and cost of healthcare.
- The *Indian Health Services* (IHS) provides comprehensive health services delivery for Native Americans and Alaskan Natives with opportunity for maximum tribal involvement in developing and managing programs to meet the health needs of these groups.
- The *National Institutes of Health* (NIH) is the principal biomedical research agency of the federal government. Its mission is to pursue knowledge to improve human health.

- The *Substance Abuse and Mental Health Services Administration* (SAMHSA) provides national leadership to ensure that knowledge, based on science and state-of-the-art practice, is effectively used for the prevention and treatment of addiction and mental disorders.

### Healthcare Financing

The Health Care Financing Agency (HCFA) was created by the Secretary of Health and Human Services in 1977 to combine under one administrative unit oversight of the Medicare program, the federal portion of the Medicaid program, and related quality assurance activities. The *Medicare program* provides health insurance coverage for people age 65 years and older, younger people who are receiving Social Security disability benefits, and a very few other persons who meet stringent criteria. The *Medicaid program* is a medical assistance program jointly financed by state and federal governments for eligible low-income individuals and recipients of Aid to Families with Dependent Children. Some states also make provisions for the needy elderly, the blind, and the disabled, who receive cash assistance under the Supplementary Security Income Program. Changes in funding and financial management of Medicare and Medicaid continue to evolve as each state becomes more responsible and accountable for oversight and quality improvement initiatives.

### Social Security Administration

The Social Security Administration (SSA) was established in 1946. In March 1995 the SSA was removed from HHS and became an independent agency. The SSA is a national program of contributory social insurance whereby employees, employers, and the self-employed pay contributions that are pooled in special trust funds.

## Administration for Children and Families and Administration on Aging

The Administration for Children and Families (ACF) was created in 1981. It is divided into the Administration on Children, Youth, and Families; the Administration of Developmental Disabilities; the Administration of Native Americans; the Office of Refugee Resettlement; and the Office of Family Assistance. The Administration on Aging (AOA) is the principal agency designated to carry out the provisions of the Older Americans Act of 1965. It is the leading agency within the HHS on all issues concerning aging.

## Making Federal Policy

The making of public policy is a complex, dynamic process that is affected by multiple variables. According to Kingdon (1984) (the Kingdon paradigm), public policy making includes setting the agenda, specifying alternatives from which a choice is to be made, making an authoritative choice among those specified alternatives, and implementing the decisions.

The three processes by which agendas are set and alternatives are specified include problem recognition, policy generation, and the political process. Each process should be viewed as an independent stream of ideas and opportunities (Calkins, Fernandopulle, & Marino, 1995). The political stream is composed of swings in national mood, administration or legislative turnover, and interest group pressure campaigns. Potential agenda items that are congruent with the current group's support (or that lack organized opposition) are more likely to rise to the agenda than those items that do not meet such conditions. According to the Kingdon paradigm, the three major players that influence federal health policy are the executive branch, Congress, and special interest groups.

Fig. 7-2 presents an overview of how a bill becomes law. In regard to healthcare and various other issues, many nurses are politically active in an effort to influence whether bills are passed or not.

How a Bill Becomes Law

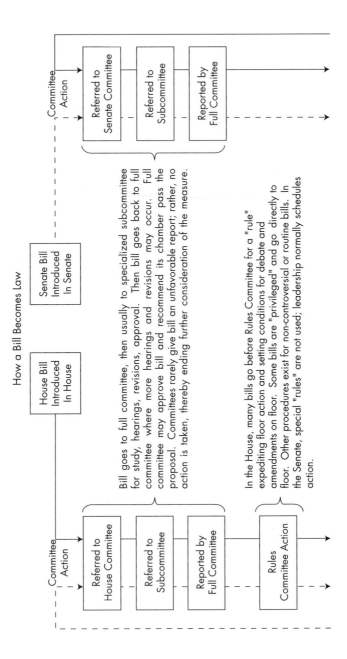

Bill goes to full committee, then usually to specialized subcommittee for study, hearings, revisions, approval. Then bill goes back to full committee where more hearings and revisions may occur. Full committee may approve bill and recommend its chamber pass the proposal. Committees rarely give bill an unfavorable report; rather, no action is taken, thereby ending further consideration of the measure.

In the House, many bills go before Rules Committee for a "rule" expediting floor action and setting conditions for debate and amendments on floor. Some bills are "privileged" and go directly to floor. Other procedures exist for non-controversial or routine bills. In the Senate, special "rules" are not used; leadership normally schedules action.

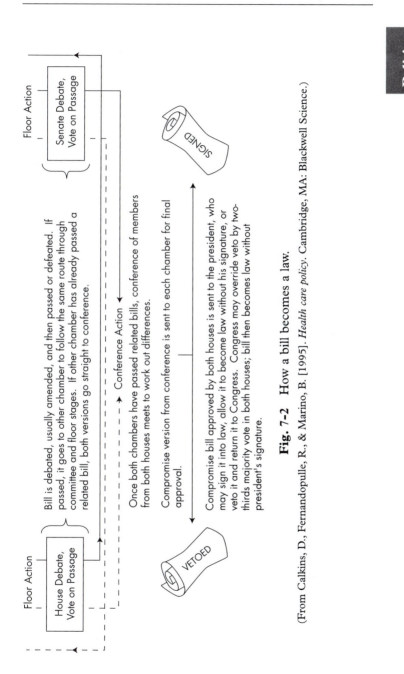

**Fig. 7-2** How a bill becomes a law.

(From Calkins, D., Fernandopulle, R., & Marino, B. [1995]. *Health care policy.* Cambridge, MA: Blackwell Science.)

## BIBLIOGRAPHY

Calkins, D., Fernandopulle, R., & Marino, B. (1995). *Health care policy.* Cambridge, MA: Blackwell Science.

Cavanaugh, D. (1985). Gamesmanship: The art of strategizing. *Journal of Nursing Administration, 4,* 39.

Kingdon, J. W. (1984). *Agendas, alternatives, and public policies.* Boston: Little, Brown.

Strasen, L. (1987). *Key business skills for nurse managers.* Philadelphia: J. B. Lippincott.

Swansburg, R. (1990). *Management and leadership for nurse managers.* Boston: Jones & Bartlett.

# Chapter 8

# Managed Care

*My obligation is to do the right thing. The rest is in God's hands.*

Martin Luther King, Jr.

## CHARACTERISTICS OF HEALTHCARE MODELS

*Managed care* is a coordinated approach to the delivery and financing of healthcare through utilization management and price/cost controls (Table 8-1).

*Capitation* is an arrangement whereby healthcare is provided according to a defined monetary amount per member. The healthcare provider assumes the financial risk if overutilization of resources occurs.

The power of capitation incentives to bring about immediate changes in physician and hospital utilization should not be underestimated. In managed care–penetrated markets, utilization changes can occur overnight. It is predicted that capitation will shortly become the dominant form of payment in the U.S. healthcare system. Under capitated contracts, physicians and hospitals receive a fixed amount per month for each health plan member, regardless of whether a member makes 10 office visits, has major surgery, or requires no services during that period.

The shift to capitation is probably the most important change in healthcare financing since the initiation of the prospective payment systems and diagnosis related groups (DRGs). According to Coile (1997), capitation is replacing other payment arrangements for the following reasons:

**231**

**Table 8-1** Healthcare Model Characteristics

| Traditional Model | New Model (Managed Care) |
|---|---|
| • Promotes volume-driven success measurements (i.e., number of admissions, number of diagnoses, number of patient days) | • Integrates health networking in an increasingly capitated environment |
| • Fosters maximum use of resources | • Promotes cost-effective care, and assesses utilization of ambulatory services |
| • Focuses on acute care as core of business | • Defines quality in terms of outcomes and community health status |
| • Equates quality with process inputs (i.e., number of services provided) | • Focuses on management of a population and taking risks |

- Purchasers can shift 100% of their financial risk to providers.
- Purchasers know exactly how much their healthcare services and benefits cost.
- Providers regain control of all monies for patient care.
- Distribution of healthcare services and payments comes under provider control.
- Purchasers can reduce their administrative overhead costs because providers take on responsibility for utilization management and quality assurance/improvement.
- Consumers know that all services are covered.
- Consumers can identify a primary physician to coordinate all their care needs.

Successful solutions to a rapidly changing healthcare challenge must be cost-effective, integrated, and rapidly deployable.

Economics will drive the future of the health industry. As price competition under managed care intensifies, the pressures to decrease the use of costly hospital care, physician services, and excessive diagnostic testing grow stronger. Market realities are beginning to affect the healthcare profession more rapidly, and changes are already evident: declining inpatient use, substitution of ambulatory care for inpatient care, primary care gatekeeping, consolidation, and integration.

## STAGES OF MANAGED CARE: ORGANIZING FOR CAPITATION AND HEALTH REFORM

The literature cites several descriptions, or stages, of progressive managed care penetration into a marketplace. The most explicit framing of managed care is described in Table 8-2.

Some individuals consider an additional stage of managed care in terms of postreform characteristics. Coile (1997) published five stages of managed care and asserts that each stage has predictable market events and strategic responses. The five stages are as follows:

- Stage 1—Can't Spell HMO
- Stage 2—Managed Care Gets Aggressive
- Stage 3—Managed Care Penetration
- Stage 4—Managed Competition
- Stage 5—Postreform

### Stage 1: Can't Spell HMO
*Characteristics*
- Health maintenance organization (HMO) penetration small
- Indemnity >30%
- Solo/small groups form open-panel independent-practice associations
- Freestanding hospital—prefers to "go it alone"
- Ambulatory services are a small percentage; do not compete with physicians
- Invest in capital spending rather than deferring capital for reserves
- Quality measured in terms of responding to JCAHO regulations

**Table 8-2** Four Stages of Managed Care (Differentiation of Progression)

| Fee-for-Service and Discounted Medicine | Managed Payment | Organized Care | Accountable Care |
|---|---|---|---|
| Inpatient delivery prevails | Inpatient utilization begins to drop | Capitation begins | Providers of care assume at-risk contracts |
| Consumer has freedom of choice | Physicians begin to sign contracts and organize | Continued drop in in-patient utilization | Primary care/gatekeeper model replaces traditional inpatient model |
| Little HMO penetration | HMO penetration widens | Large physician groups emerge | Large numbers of hospitals affiliate, merge, or close |
| Hospital is at center of delivery model | Hospital begins to affiliate/merge | HMO penetration widens to smaller markets | HMO penetration dominates market |

VHA Information Technology Study, 1995.

### Stage 2: Managed Care Gets Aggressive
*Characteristics*
- HMO penetration remains <15%; however, HMO contracts with primary care physician (PCP) groups
- Early capitation contracting; majority provider payments with discounts
- Employers form coalitions and share data
- Small medical groups merge without "walls"
- Ambulatory care remains <20%
- Early cost containment
- Quality measured by benchmarking

### Stage 3: Managed Care Penetration
*Characteristics*
- HMO penetration increasing; closed physician-hospital organization (PHO)/physician groups
- Begin direct contracting
- Single-specialty groups; increase of primary care groups
- Mergers and expansion of systems
- Profits 2% to 4%; necessary to restructure staff and management
- Quality measured through patient-focused care initiatives

### Stage 4: Managed Competition
*Characteristics*
- HMO penetration 25% to 40% with regional networks
- Indemnity <5% with point-of-service (POS) plans
- Employers use purchasing coalitions
- Ambulatory care >40% and increasing; experiencing excess inpatient beds
- Profits 1% to 2%; necessary to reengineer patient care
- Quality measured through utilization of clinical paths/ outcomes

Managed Care

**Stage 5: Postreform**

*Characteristics*

- HMO penetration >40% with foundation/equity models
- Indemnity target 0%; strong POS networks
- Ambulatory care >50%; continuum of care developing
- Physician mega-groups; equity and staff models
- Clinical costs management
- Quality measured through outcomes/patient ratings

## DELIVERY SYSTEM RESTRUCTURING

1. Patient care will need to be managed and delivered with fixed dollars in a manner that produces superior clinical outcomes and excellent customer service.
2. At every level, caps and incentives will encourage the use of the least costly provider that can give quality care.
3. The primary care focus on prevention and wellness will require providers to understand and capture the psychosocial and behavioral aspects of compliance and personal responsibility.
4. Provider networks will increasingly use nurse practitioners to service primary care entry points.

## What Are Managed Care Companies Looking For?

- Responsiveness and the ability to customize services to meet member needs
- Quality clinical programs with above-average outcomes
- One-stop shopping (vertical integration); a seamless system
- Experience in serving Medicare and non-Medicare market of people of all ages
- Competitive and outcome-oriented pricing
- Marketing ability and commitment
- Internal case management
- Attitude of partnership
- Understanding and support of managed care philosophy

## What Do Patients Want?

- Caring and concerned staff
- Competent caregivers
- Clear and timely communication
- Cleanliness
- Quiet atmosphere
- Services:
  —Choices
  —No waiting
  —Streamlined admissions
  —Expedited discharge

## What Do Physicians Want?

- Competent care for their patients
- Streamlined access to hospital (e.g., admissions, surgery, scheduling)
- Nurse availability
- Information readily available (e.g., charts, test results)

## CHARACTERISTICS OF THE EMERGING HEALTH SYSTEM (PEW Health Professions Commission, 1993)

1. *Orientation toward health:* greater emphasis on prevention and wellness; greater expectation of individual responsibility for healthy behaviors
2. *Population perspective:* new attention to risk factors affecting substantial segments of the community, including issues of access and the physical and social environment
3. *Intensive use of information:* reliance on information systems to provide complete, easily assimilated patient information, as well as ready access to relevant information on current practice
4. *Focus on the consumer:* expectation and encouragement of patient partnerships in decisions related to treatment, facilitated by availability of complete information on outcomes and evaluated in part by patient satisfaction

5. *Knowledge of treatment outcomes:* emphasis on determination of the most effective treatment under different conditions and dissemination of this information to those involved in treatment decisions

6. *Constrained resources:* a pervasive concern over increasing costs, coupled with expanded use of mechanisms to control or limit available expenditures

7. *Coordination of services:* increased integration of providers with a concomitant emphasis on teams to improve efficiency and effectiveness across all settings

8. *Reconsideration of human values:* careful assessment of the balance between the expanding capability of technology and the need for humane treatment

9. *Expectations of accountability:* growing scrutiny by a larger variety of payers, consumers, and regulators, coupled with more formally defined performance expectations

10. *Growing interdependence:* further integration of domestic issues of health, education, and public safety, combined with a growing awareness of the importance of U.S. healthcare in a global context

## PROFESSIONAL ATTRIBUTES REQUIRED FOR MANAGED CARE ORGANIZATION SURVIVAL

To pursue a career in a managed care organization (MCO), one must possess, or be able to learn, the characteristics of a team player, exhibiting the following traits (Reres, 1996):

- *Flexibility.* Flexibility is not necessarily the ability to bend. More important, it is equated with openness (being open to new ideas, research findings, trends, customer needs; exposing what one does not know; changing from independence to interdependence). Flexibility then leads to versatility (not easily acquired by individuals who value predictability).

- *Focus.* In work teams one must stay focused on the here-and-now, constantly learning and building on new concepts and ideas. Focusing has the added benefits of

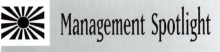

## Management Spotlight

- Be a good sport:
  - Promote harmony.
  - Play fair . . . show respect for others instead of putting someone down.
  - Demonstrate humility . . . big enough to admit mistake and say "I'm sorry."
- If peers are negative, the reactive person becomes negative with them.
- Proactive people are value-driven. They remain positive and give a quality performance regardless of circumstances or attitudes around them.

Data from Pritchett, P. (1997). *The team member handbook for team work*. Dallas: Pritchett & Associates.

diminishing stress during periods of organizational change and fostering higher productivity.

- *Energy.* Energy adds positive attitudes and vitality to the organization. Negativity not only thwarts results but also brews frustration and saps energy.
- *Security.* Formerly, security meant lifetime employment in a given organization. In a managed care environment roles change as markets and community needs change, and new systems evolve. Security in a managed care organization is equated to marketability. To be prepared for role changes, one must continually add new skills and diversity.
- *Collegiality.* Learn from colleagues. It is important to make dedicated efforts to the corporate health of the organization.
- *Valued identification.* An individual needs to choose an MCO with basic values similar to his or her own. Determine whether or not the MCO is congruent with your core values.

## MODELS OF PATIENT CARE DELIVERY
### Team Nursing

*Team nursing* is a delivery model in which the registered nurse (RN) is utilized as a team leader for a group of professional and paraprofessional staff to care for a group of patients. The team can vary in structure, skill level, and size. The team constituents and the use of those constituents will also vary from department to department and between organizations.

The team leader is responsible for assessing patient care needs, prioritizing and delegating the interventions required to meet those needs, and evaluating patient care activities for the shift. Depending on variables such as acuity and staffing fluctuations, the team leader may be required to modify patient assignments and delegation of interventions to accommodate the changing needs of the patient. Delegation of interventions to other team members must be made in accordance with the skill level and legal scope of practice for each member. In addition, the competency documentation for each team member must be easily accessed by the team leader to make appropriate assignments. The key to delegation and team nursing is communication among the team members and the patient/family.

According to Marrelli (1997), the strengths of the team nursing model are efficiencies in care and costs, as opposed to other models such as total patient care and primary nursing. Weaknesses include limited accountability (because everyone is accountable) and the costs associated with the daily needs for conference time with the group. Perception by the patient is that continuity of care is limited since several caregivers are involved during one shift. An assumption regarding team nursing is that care may become fragmented in this model as compared to a total patient approach.

### Total Patient Care

*Total patient care* is a nursing care delivery pattern in which the RN or licensed practical nurse (LPN) is responsible for providing all the care to a smaller group of patients. Even though an LPN is often used in this model, all LPNs and other paraprofessional nursing staff must be supervised by an RN. The strengths of total patient care are that the patient care assignments are smaller and, theoretically, the nurse has a more extensive knowledge base of assigned patients. Therefore patient care is perceived by the patient and RN as comprehensive and less fragmented. The weaknesses of the model are higher costs and the fact that continuity is limited when one nurse covers for another.

## Primary Nursing

*Primary nursing* is a model in which the RN is given the assignment of coordinating all the care for a group of patients—for the total hospitalization of those patients 24 hours per day (Marrelli, 1997). This nurse, called the primary nurse, may also provide some care for the patients and delegate the rest. An associate nurse cares for the patient in the absence of the primary nurse; however, the associate follows the plan of care initiated by the primary nurse. Marrelli further asserts that the primary nurse is accountable for the outcomes of care and care planning and for subsequent documentation.

The strengths of primary nursing are higher patient satisfaction, continuity of care, and perception of a higher quality of care provided. The weakness of primary nursing is related to fiscal management. Primary nursing is more costly than team or functional nursing because of the dependence on a greater number of RNs and the nonproductive time involved in care planning.

## Modular Nursing

*Modular nursing* is similar to team nursing in that a nurse is assigned the nursing care for a group of patients in relationship to the geographical location or logistics of the clinical

Managed Care

area. The nurse is assigned a paraprofessional (LPN or nursing assistant [NA]). Teams in modular nursing are smaller and facilitate closer monitoring of the patients by the RN than in the team nursing model. Modular nursing uses fewer RNs and thus is less costly than primary nursing. However, modular nursing is less efficient and more costly than team nursing.

### Functional Nursing

*Functional nursing* is a patient care delivery model in which staff are given interventions to perform in accordance with their individual scope of practice and level of competency. Continuity of care is strained because many caregivers are involved with care of the patient. An example of functional nursing is when one nurse gives medication, another nurse does all the dressing changes on the shift, and a third nurse does all the charting and related duties.

From a financial standpoint, the functional model uses different skill levels and is considered to be the most efficient and least costly delivery model (Marrelli, 1997). From the patient's perspective, however, the functional model is task-oriented and requires multiple caregivers to meet the needs of one patient. From the employee's perspective, the functional model provides the least challenge.

### Case Management

*Case management* models represent a newer generation of primary nursing. The case manager is responsible for managing the care of a group of patients across all clinical areas within a current hospitalization. There are several case management models evolving, and the case manager is not always a nurse. Physicians, social workers, discharge planners, and dietitians are examples of professionals working in hospitals who have been known to serve as case managers. Protocols and the treatment plan are developed by the healthcare team. Subsequent outcomes management is also monitored by the team.

Since case management models differ, so does the financial impact. The utilization of protocols and clinical pathways greatly reduces cost in terms of reduced length of stay and fewer delayed discharges. Case management is viewed by many authors as the nursing care delivery model of the future, especially as managed care environments evolve and emphasis is placed on the continuum of care.

Because healthcare needs are different from unit to unit, frequently there are variations of each of the models utilized. According to Marrelli (1997), factors that should be considered when selecting a patient care delivery model include:

- Vision, philosophy, and core values of the patient care nursing service
- Numbers, skill mix, competency, and quality of available nursing personnel
- Customer demands/desires vs. marketplace competition
- Turnover rate and retention status of nursing employees
- Financial status of the organization; budgetary resource and salary allocation

### Case management through differentiated practice

The roles in this model are selected by the individual nurse based on competency, desire, and education. The roles that form the foundation are associate nurse, primary nurse, and advanced practice nurse (Cohen, 1996).

The *associate nurse* is responsible for patient care within a determined amount of time, such as a single shift, during a patient episode of illness. The *primary nurse* is responsible for coordinating patient care from admission to discharge during an episode of illness. The primary nurse will coordinate resources and discharge planning. The *advanced practice nurse* (*clinical nurse specialist* or *nurse practitioner*) is responsible for coordinating the care throughout the continuum of care and across all settings. The clinical nurse specialist also fulfills the traditional role components of expert clinician, consultant, educator, researcher, and manager.

## Professionally Advanced Team Model

The *professionally advanced team model* (ProAct) has been developed through redesign processes in response to reengineering initiatives set forth by efficiency efforts in managed care. In this model two distinct nurse roles are defined. The primary nurse manages a group of patients; care is delegated according to skill mix and scope of practice. The clinical manager manages a designated caseload during the entire hospital stay. This model, much like case management models, utilizes clinical and nonclinical support persons.

## Partners in Care

*Partners in care* can be compared to primary and modular nursing. In this model paraprofessionals coupled with an RN act as partners in delivering care to a group of assigned patients. Interventions with the partnerships can vary depending on skill level and caregiver interests and preferences. In its purest form the "partners" work the same shift and the same schedule to give care to patients.

## Patient-Centered Care

Taking cues from the external environment of healthcare changes, many hospitals have transformed traditional operations into customer-oriented, patient-centered care delivery models. Through redesign efforts the focus currently involves an analysis and redefinition of all activities involved with patients. The focus for patient care is a high-quality, cost-effective multidisciplinary approach.

Depending on the unique characteristics and needs of individual organizational systems, the work redesign in a patient-centered care model is implemented by using nontraditional roles to provide tasks or interventions for patient care. An example of patient care delivery patterns is the use of a phlebotomist or an environmental service employee in the nursing assistant role. Many systems also incorporate the nontraditional employee into a unit-specific role, with the clinical nurse manager supervising and evaluating that individual.

Fig. 8-1 depicts the critical aspects of a patient-focused care initiative, balancing quality and cost-effectiveness outcomes. In addition, the chart shows that the overall goals are directed toward customer satisfaction (patient/family, physician, employee).

## IMPLEMENTING CRITICAL PATHWAYS

*Outcome-based practice* is a combination of the result and the framework for case management. Outcomes are mutually agreed on by all disciplines and are reflected in the documentation pathway. Outcomes-based practice is the umbrella for care management, case management, resource management, and program management.

*Case management* is a coordinated care effort that is patient centered, outcome oriented, and multidisciplinarily managed. According to Mundt (1996), the key elements to case management are client-centered approach, coordination of care and services across a variety of settings, outcome oriented, resource efficient, and collaborative and cooperative. *Care management* (The Living at Home/Block Nursing Program) is a community program to provide service coordination to enable the elderly to remain healthy and remain in their homes (Jamieson, 1996). *Resource management* is the process of identifying and negotiating resources for the patient. This includes everything from preeligibility screening to postdischarge needs. *Program management* encompasses the construction of a formal system to deliver care and services to a specified population of patients with similar needs. This includes consistent availability of services, not access to services.

*Critical/clinical pathways* have many names: practice guidelines, care tracks, CareMaps, care process models, collaborative paths, and anticipated recovery paths—to name a few

## PATIENT-FOCUSED CARE INITIATIVE

| STAFF SATISFACTION | PATIENT SATISFACTION | PHYSICIAN SATISFACTION |
|---|---|---|
| Qualified staff available | Involvement in Plan of Care | Staff available to discuss goals and make rounds |
| Involved with unit-based CQI, standards, etc. | Courteous, responsive staff (nursing, RT, Lab, etc.) | Timely reports, results on charts and available |
| Working to max of job descriptions | Clean, safe, quite environment | Communication systems exist that minimize disruptions to office practice, but meet IP needs |
| Feel empowered to make changes | Understandable bills | Tests, procedures, etc. completed in a timely manner |
| Collaboration with MDs and others (critical paths, etc.) | Thorough education before discharge | |
| Bias toward action with CQI focus | Appropriate discharge follow-up | |
| Accountability-based practice | Smooth admitting, discharge, and/or transfer process | |
| | MD available and informative | |

| | Quality/ Cost Effective Outcome |
|---|---|
| Appropriate utilization of Lab, X-ray, ECGs | Case management of difficult patients |
| Discharge within established DRG LOS | Staff aware of "critical path" and variances early |
| Appropriate utilization of staff | RNs responsible/accountable for coordination/implementation of Plan of Care with other disciplines |
| Systems designed to meet patients' needs efficiently | Vigorous attention to ambulation, skin care, and patient safety issues |
| Appropriate services are unit-based | Transcription of orders and implementation of same is accurate and timely |
| Appropriate use of technology (Pharmacy, ATH's) | Evaluation/intervention of any delays in treatment or problems that affect LOS/outcomes |
| LOS cost | Low infection role |
| COMPLICATION RATE | Low complication role |
| LOW COST | |

**Fig. 8-1**  Patient-Focused Care Initiative.

Managed Care

(*Action Tips* box and Fig. 8-2). Critical pathways are developed for a defined homogeneous patient population in which a multidisciplinary team cares for the patient throughout an episode of care. In addition, critical pathways are used to:

- Coordinate, deliver, monitor, and evaluate care concurrently
- Create a multidisciplinary standard of practice
- Articulate critical incidents and variance reporting
- Allow for aggregate data analysis of care episode
- Promote interdisciplinary collaboration, communication, and information

General goals for the implementation of critical pathways in an organization include the following:

- Promote coordination and continuity of care
- Promote collaboration of care planning and implementation among the multidisciplines
- Forecast expected clinical outcomes
- Monitor utilization of resources and lengths of stay
- Change practice based on outcomes research (clinical and fiscal outcomes)
- Streamline documentation
- Provide access to multidisciplinary information/communication
- Promote patient and family involvement

The following factors should be considered when selecting DRGs to be case managed.

- High cost, high volume, extended length of stay, or known inappropriate use of resources
- High interest, high market value
- High potential for service delivery fragmentation
- High incidence of readmissions
- High variation in clinical/financial outcome
- Physician interest

**Negotiation Tactics** (Fuller, 1990)

- No matter what you are bargaining for, always perform a "what if" analysis of alternatives before starting.

CRITICAL PATHWAY IMPLEMENTATION CHECKLIST

Unit: _____          Expected GO-LIVE Date: _____

| Steps | Respon-sible Persons | Date Due | Date Com-pleted |
|---|---|---|---|
| 1. Choose DRG | | | |
| 2. Research cost and LOS (per physician); generate report to share | | | |
| 3. Obtain HCFA/payor Mean LOS and reimbursement | | | |
| 4. Determine team members (all disciplines should participate in pathway development). | | | |
| 5. Develop the pathway<br>• Chart review for practice pattern (10-12 charts)<br>• Literature review for existing pathways | | | |
| 6. Complete<br>• Preprinted physician orders<br>• Patient's plan of care<br>• Patient education and handouts<br>• Review by staff | | | |
| 7. Develop financial pathway from final draft, if appropriate | | | |
| 8. Meet with key physicians for review/approval and to educate | | | |
| 9. Staff preparation/buy in<br>• Identify go-live date<br>• Plan inservices on documentation, and specific PI plan | | | |
| 10. Go-Live<br>• Test critical pathway for 24-hours before go-live<br>• Case managers, educators, and implementation team available as resources on go-live date<br>• Weekly meetings with case managers<br>• Follow-up focus group meetings every 2 weeks and then every month to make revisions. | | | |
| 11. Begin data collection for Performance Improvement plan; Determine monthly variance reporting mechanism | | | |

Modified from: Mount Carmel Medical Center, Columbus, OH

**Managed Care**

**Fig. 8-2**   Critical Pathway Implementation Checklist.

## Action Tips

### CRITICAL/CLINICAL PATHWAY DEVELOPMENT

- *Step 1:* Select DRGs to be case managed.
- *Step 2:* Identify specific physicians to participate based on admitting patterns, expertise, or expressed interest.
- *Step 3:* Provide educational sessions for the clinical pathway development team based on experience and knowledge level of pathways.
- *Step 4:* Write the plan of care collaboratively with all the disciplines. Plan of care will include consults, assessments, interventions and treatments, discharge planning, and patient/family education.
- *Step 5:* Develop measures of conformance and outcomes.
- *Step 6:* Pilot the critical pathway. Staff education efforts may need to be repeated during this time. Communicate.
- *Step 7:* Go live! Implement the pathway (Fig. 8-2).
- *Step 8:* Evaluate the critical pathway: Use the individual organization's performance improvement program/plan design. Determine who is responsible for variance tracking and reporting. Outcome variations should be documented and reviewed daily to address patient problems actively. Institute continuous improvement.

- Know what your terminal objectives are and what you expect to be offered in return.
- Picture yourself in the other person's (or company's) position, and imagine what they want and for what they would likely settle.
- Establish a well-planned fall-back position. Decide what concessions can be made to reach an agreement.
- Ensure that everyone participating in the negotiation is briefed so that there are no surprises.

**INTEGRATED CLINICAL PATHWAY**

DIABETES AND INSULIN MANAGEMENT FOR ADULTS
Physician Group:
Attending MD:
DRG: 294
Primary RN: ______
Date Reviewed by MD/RN/Patient: ______
Advance Directive: Yes____ No____
Code Status: ______

**MEDICAL HISTORY**

| Admit Date | ICU Date | Transfer Date | Allergies: |
|---|---|---|---|
| Present problem: | | | Surgical & special procedures: |
| Past history: | | | |

**Physician Consults:**

| Date | Physician | Reason | First visit | Signed off |
|---|---|---|---|---|
| | | | | |

**Phone Numbers:**
Name ______
Relationship ______
Home ______
Work ______
Name ______
Relationship ______
Home ______
Work ______

DISCHARGE PLANNING

| Discharge Destination | Initiated D/C Plan Date/Initial | D/C Outcome Date/Initial | Community Services | Initiated D/C Plan Date/Initial | D/C Outcome Date/Initial | Transportation | Initiated D/C Plan Date/Initial | D/C Outcome Date/Initial |
|---|---|---|---|---|---|---|---|---|
| Home alone/family | / | / | Dept. social services | / | / | Family | / | / |
| Home w/ | / | / | Senior companion | / | / | Wheelchair service | / | / |
| Home w/home health ____ | / | / | Homemaker | / | / | Paratransit | / | / |
| Home w/public health nurse __ | / | / | Respite care | / | / | Ambulance | / | / |
| Nursing home, skilled ____ | / | / | Meals on wheels | / | / | Indian health services | / | / |
| Nursing home, intermediate__ | / | / | Lifeline | / | / | State penitentiary | / | / |
| Nursing home, | | | HEARTH | / | / | Other ______ | / | / |
| assisted living | / | / | Hospice | / | / | | | |
| Rehab ______ | / | / | Wellness center ____ | / | / | Equipment | Date/Initial | Date/Initial |
| Swing bed: ______ | / | / | Cardiac rehab ____ | / | / | Home oxygen | / | / |
| VA hospital | / | / | Vascular rehab ____ | / | / | Home IV therapy ____ | / | / |
| Hospice cottage | / | / | Support group ____ | | | Assistive devices ____ | / | / |
| State penitentiary | / | / | ______ | / | / | ______ | | |
| Hotel ______ | / | / | Other ______ | / | / | Other: ______ | / | / |
| Other______ | / | / | | | | | | |

Initials/Signature: ____/______ ____/______
____/______ ____/______ ____/______

OFF PATHWAY ☐ YES
DATE ____/____/____

**If pathway discontinued, chart summation note as to reason why discontinued.**
01/95 CHART FORM



**Fig. 8-3** Integrated Clinical Pathway.
(Courtesy Sioux Valley Hospital, Sioux Falls, SD.)

*Continued*

- When possible, use the "home court advantage" for meeting places. The next best place would be somewhere neutral to both parties.
- Never negotiate with someone who does not have the authority to reach an agreement.
- Keep emotions in check. Sometimes experienced negotiators attempt to cause frustration so that mistakes are made.
- Suggest a coffee break if things are not going in a favorable direction. The break gives time to rethink strategies.
- Confirm all agreements in writing as soon as possible.
- If an agreement is not reached, if possible, let the other party make the first contact.

Managed Care

| DAY/DATE | Day Admit    Date _____ | Day 1    Date _____ |
|---|---|---|
| CONSULTS | Contact diabetes educator (pager 1359)<br>Dietician | |
| LABS<br>X-RAY<br>OTHER | Daily    FBS, 11, 4, 10 (one touch)<br>          CBC, UA, lytes | Daily    FBS, 11, 4, 10 (one touch)<br>          Can use patient's meter if readings are<br>          within 20% of labs x 3 |
| TREATMENTS/<br>PULMONARY | Order glucose meter | |
| MEDICATIONS/<br>IVs | Insulin | Insulin |
| NUTRITION | _____ cal ADA | _____ cal ADA |
| ACTIVITY/PT<br>SAFETY | Up ad lib | Up ad lib |
| DISCHARGE<br>PLANNING | Complete assessment tool<br>Initiate data base | Review data base<br>Discuss home arrangements |
| NURSING DX/<br>INTERDISCIPLINARY<br>FOCUS | Knowledge                        Anxiety<br>Potential hypoglycemia        Hyperglycemia<br>Fluid volume | Knowledge                        Anxiety<br>Potential hypoglycemia        Hyperglycemia<br>Fluid volume: resolve |
| KEY NURSING<br>ACTIVITIES/<br>TEACHING | Record B.S. on diabetes flow sheet<br>VS routine, I & O, Wt<br>Assess LOC and S&S hypo/hyper q 4 hrs<br>Push fluids<br>      Education emphasis<br>      1. Provide diabetes folder/film list ___<br>      2. B & S hypoglycemia/hyperglycemia ___<br><br>KEY<br>A = Pt/family verbalize understanding<br>B = Pt/family need reinforcement<br>C = Pt/family not available | VS routine, I & O<br>Assess LOC and S & S hypo/hyper q 4 hrs<br>Push fluids<br>Record BS on flow sheet<br>Attends DB classes/watches films<br>      Education emphasis<br>      1. Blood glucose meter ___<br>      2. Hypoglycemia ___<br>      3. What is diabetes ___<br>      4. Nutrition ___<br>      5. Reinforce education ___<br><br>KEY<br>A = Pt/family verbalize understanding<br>B = Pt/family need reinforcement<br>C = Pt/family not available |
| KEY PATIENT<br>OUTCOMES | 1. Verbalizes S & S of hypoglycemia<br>2. Begin looking at diabetes folder<br>3. Assessment within normal limits (WNL) for patient | 1. Demonstrates One Touch meter<br>2. Verbalizes basic understanding of diabetes,<br>   hypoglycemia and nutrition<br>3. Assessment WNL for patient; no s/s of<br>   hypo/hyperglycemia |
| SHIFT<br>RN SIGNATURE | D.<br>N. | D.<br>N. |
| INITIALS/<br>SIGNATURE | _____ /_____<br>_____ /_____ | _____ /_____<br>_____ /_____ |

**Fig. 8-3**    Cont'd. Integrated Clinical Pathway.

## ETHICS AND MANAGED CARE

Healthcare organizations are beginning to incorporate ethical guidelines into managed care contracting. These guidelines help challenge insurance companies and HMOs to cover the needs of the underserved populations. According to Appleby (1996), incorporating ethics into business decisions has stymied healthcare executives across the country. He states that now both the press and consumers keep a wary eye for ethical breaches. Whether they are fulfilling a mission or just trying to avoid bad publicity, managed care groups are facing tough new challenges with deals and decision-making based

| Day 2    Date _____ | Day 3    Date _____ | Day 4    Date _____ |
|---|---|---|
| | | DISHCARGE |
| Daily   FBS, 11, 4, 10 (one touch)<br>Can use patient's meter if readings<br>are within 20% of labs x 3 | Daily   FBS, 11, 4, 10 (one touch)<br>Can use patient's meter if readings<br>are within 20% of labs x 3 | Daily   FBS, 11, 4, 10 (one touch)<br>Can use patient's meter if readings<br>are within 20% of labs x 3 |
| | | |
| Insulin | Insulin | Insulin |
| _____ cal ADA | _____ cal ADA | _____ cal ADA |
| Up ad lib | Up ad lib | Up ad lib |
| Review plans, revise as needed | Review plans, revise as needed<br>Confirm home arrangements | Finalize discharge plans |
| Knowledge                         Anxiety<br>Potential hypoglycemia<br>Hyperglycemia: resolve | Knowledge<br>Potential hypoglycemia<br>Anxiety | Knowledge: resolve<br>Potential hypoglycemia: resolve<br>Anxiety: resolve |
| VS routine, I & O<br>Assess LOC and S & S hypo/hyper q 4 hrs<br>Push fluids<br>Record BS on flow sheet<br>Attends DB classes/watches films<br>Pt administers own pm insulin<br>　Education emphasis<br>　1. Insulin/medication ___<br>　2. Nutrition ___<br>　3. Exercise ___<br>　4. Emotions ___<br>　5. Reinforce education ___<br><br>　　　KEY<br>　A = Pt/family verbalize understanding<br>　B = Pt/family need reinforcement<br>　C = Pt/family not available | Pt administers own insulin<br>VS routine, I & O<br>Assess LOC and S & S hypo/hyper q 4 hrs<br>Push fluids<br>Record BS on flow sheet<br>Attends DB classes/watches films<br>　Education<br>　1. Sick day/ketoacidosis ___<br>　2. Diabetes complications ___<br>　3. Home management, community<br>　　resources and accessing care ___<br>　4. Reinforce education ___<br><br>　　　KEY<br>　A = Pt/family verbalize understanding<br>　B = Pt/family need reinforcement<br>　C = Pt/family not available | Pt administers own insulin<br>Reinforce education<br>Finalize discharge teaching and provide<br>　written instructions<br><br><br>Education<br>1. Community resources and<br>　accessing care ___<br>2. Home management ___<br><br>　　　KEY<br>　A = Pt/family verbalize understanding<br>　B = Pt/family need reinforcement<br>　C = Pt/family not available |
| 1. Demonstrates & administers insulin<br>2. Verbalizes understanding of diet<br>3. Verbalizes understanding of effect<br>　of exercise<br>4. Demonstrates glucose meter<br>5. Verbalizes feelings regarding diabetes<br>6. Assessment WNL for patient, no s/s of<br>　hypo/hyperglycemia | 1. Demonstrates & administers insulin<br>2. Discuss sick day management/<br>　ketoacidosis<br>3. Verbalizes measures to prevent<br>　complications<br>4. Verbalizes home management of diet,<br>　exercise, insulin, and B9M and hygiene<br>5. Demonstrates glucose meter<br>6. Assessment WNL for patient, no s/s of<br>　hypo/hyperglycemia | 1. Demonstrates & administers insulin<br>2. Verbalizes understanding of discharge<br>　instructions<br>3. Demonstrates glucose meter<br>4. Assessment WNL for patient, no s/s of<br>　hypo/hyperglycemia |
| D.<br>N. | D.<br>N. | D.<br>N. |
| _____/_____<br>_____/_____ | _____/_____<br>_____/_____ | _____/_____<br>_____/_____ |

| Special Orders | | | |
|---|---|---|---|
| KEY<br>1. Initialed in red = ordered<br>2. Black line = not ordered<br>3. Circled in black = exception | _____ | _____ | _____ |
| | _____ | _____ | _____ |
| | _____ | _____ | _____ |

**Fig. 8-3**   Cont'd. Integrated Clinical Pathway

on the often emotional and controversial concepts related to ethics. Examples of ethical guidelines that have been incorporated into contracts are as follows:

- HMOs that subscribe to the guidelines agree not to market themselves in a way that would discourage the enrollment of less desirable insurance risks, such as the poor and the disabled.
- General principles of delivery emphasize that patients will receive affordable, quality, and accessible care.

There has been a growing awareness that, with the significant evolutions taking place within the healthcare industry, the full range of religious, social, and ethical teachings on the changing conditions of healthcare have surfaced. Ethical guidelines and ethics committee interviews are part of the contract review process for the nonsecular healthcare organizations. It is important to ensure that contracts are pertinent to the specific conflicting issues, in addition to upholding the mission.

Organizationally, managed care delivery systems can be viewed as a series of relationships based on negotiated arrangements. They are subject to standards of accountability and require clarity of purpose and continuous communication (Grazier, 1998). Financially, managed care requires the implementation of sound fiscal principles, an accounting for costs, and the ability to match anticipated revenues with anticipated expenses. Managed care requires epidemiological data on the sources and patterns of utilization and illness.

The public has the right to ask about the ethics of how and why decisions are made in regard to the healthcare providers and the services selected for a particular health plan. Clear ethical principles can be a foundation for decision making at all levels. The Allina Health System published its principles, which can be applied to any health plan or system to guide practice and decision making (Ehlen & Sprenger, 1998). The principles in Allina's plan include:
- Stewardship
- Respect and caring
- Confidentiality
- Advocacy
- Honesty

## MANAGED CARE CONTINUUM MODELS

Managed care is often thought of as a continuum of models. The models are generally classified as follows (Wopler, 1995):

1. Indemnity insurance (with precertification, mandatory second opinion, and large-case management) (High percentage of clients are case managed.)
2. Service plan (with precertification, mandatory second opinion and large-case management)
3. Preferred provider organization (PPO)
4. Point-of-service (POS)
5. Health maintenance organization (HMO)
   - Open panel
     —Individual practice association (IPA)
     —Direct contract
   - Network model
   - Closed panel
     —Group model
     —Staff model

## TYPES OF HEALTH PLANS (WOPLER, 1995)
### Government Programs

A great percentage of healthcare in the United States is provided or financed by federal and state government. Programs include Medicare for the elderly and disabled and Medicaid for the poor. There are programs for active-duty military and their families and veterans. Civilian health programs are offered by the PHS. These programs may incorporate some or all features of managed care.

### Traditional Insurance

"Traditional" insurance is rapidly becoming nontraditional. It consists of two basic types: indemnity insurance and service plans.

- *Indemnity insurance.* This type protects (indemnifies) the insured against financial losses from medical expenses. Usually restrictions are involved, and benefits are generally subject to deductibles. Costs for this type of healthcare coverage have been escalating faster than for any other type of health plan. As the costs rise, more people are moving into managed care.

- *Service plan.* This term applies primarily to plans such as those of Blue Cross and Blue Shield. In service plans there are generally few restrictions on providers, who agree to sign a contract with the plan. The plan agrees to reimburse the provider directly; the provider agrees to accept the plan's fee structure. Service plans usually have discounts. Their major advantage over indemnity insurance is the presence of the provider contracts and the reimbursement models.

## PPO: Preferred Provider Organization

PPOs are similar to service plans with some differences: the total panel of providers is somewhat reduced. Reimbursement is generally the same as that of a service plan; however, usually the discounts are generous. Precertification, large-case management, and second opinion are usually components.

## HMO: Health Maintenance Organization

The majority of HMOs manage utilization and quality. HMOs are generally open paneled or closed paneled. However, a third type, the network model, is becoming increasingly popular.

- *Open panel plan.* The HMO contracts with private physicians to see members in the provider's own office. Two broad categories are IPAs and direct models.
- *Closed panel plan.* The HMO uses physicians whose practice is confined to the HMO.
- *Network model.* The HMO contracts with several large multispecialty medical groups.

## POS: Point of Service

These plans combine features of HMOs with those of traditional insurance. Members may choose which system to use at the point when they obtain the service.

## BIBLIOGRAPHY

Appleby, C. (1996). True values. *Hospitals and Health Networks, 70*(30), 20-26.

Capuano, T. (1995). Clinical pathways: Practical approaches, positive outcomes. *Nursing Management, 26*(10), 34-37.

Cerne, F., & Montague, J. (1994). Capacity crisis. *Hospital and Health Networks,* OCT, (11) 30-40.

Cohen, E.L. (1996). *Nurse case management in the 21st century.* St. Louis: Mosby.

Coile, R. (1997). *The five stages of managed care: Strategies for providers, HMOs, and suppliers.* Management Series, American College of Healthcare Executives. Chicago: Health Administration Press.

DeBack, V., & Cohen, E. (1996). The new practice environment. In E.L. Cohen, *Nurse case management in the 21st century.* St. Louis: Mosby.

DeWoody, S., & Price, J. (1994). A systems approach to multidimensional critical paths. *Nursing Management, 25*(11), 47-51.

Ehlen, K., & Sprenger, G. (1998). Ethics and decision making in healthcare. *Journal of Healthcare Management, 43*(3), 219-221.

Fuller, G. (1990). *The supervisor's portable answer book.* Englewood Cliffs, NJ: Prentice-Hall.

Grazier, K. (1998). Looking closely at managed care. *Journal of Healthcare Management, 43*(1), 1-5.

Jamieson, M. (1996). Grass roots efforts: Nurses involved in the political process. In E.L. Cohen, *Nurse case management in the 21st century.* St. Louis: Mosby.

Kleeb, T. (1995). *Pathways and algorithms.* Catholic Health Corporation.

Marrelli, T.M. (1997). *The nurse manager's survival guide: Practical answers to everyday problems* (2nd ed.). St. Louis: Mosby.

Marwick, C. (1996). Effect of managed care felt in every medical field. *JAMA, 276*(10), 768-769.

McKenzie, C., Torkelson, N., & Holt, M. (1989). Care and cost: Nursing case management improves both. *Nursing Management, 20*(10), 38-42.

Mundt, M. (1996). Key elements of nurse case management in curricula. In E.L. Cohen, *Nurse case management in the 21st century.* St. Louis: Mosby.

PEW Health Professions Commission (1993). *Health professions education for the future: Schools in service to the nation,* San Fransico: PEW Memorial Trust.

Reres, M. (1996). *Managed care: Managing the process.* Glencoe, MO: National Professional Education Institute.

Wopler, L. (1995). *Health care administration: Principles, practices, structure, and delivery.* Rockville, MD: Aspen Publishers.

# Chapter 9

# Competency-Based Education

Vivien Jutsum

*If you believe your employees can do anything. . .they can!
Give them the opportunity to experience the same feeling of
achievement that ignites your enthusiasm.*

*Roey Kirk*

The traditional approach to measuring nursing staff competence has been the use of credentials such as licenses and specialty certifications established through knowledge-based
testing, usually with multiple-choice type tests. However,
more recently, there has been a new focus on measuring competence by evaluating actual performance—either on the job
or in a simulated situation. This focus, initiated by del Bueno
in the 1970s, continues today. To a large extent it is driven by
the Joint Commission on Accreditation of Healthcare Organizations (JCAHO), which since 1992 has addressed the
need to evaluate performance in delivering patient care and
to define clearly the process by which this evaluation is
achieved. Since 1995 JCAHO has increased its expectations
to include the evaluation of competence for all healthcare
employees, not just nursing, stating "processes are designed
to ensure that the competence of all staff members is
assessed, maintained, demonstrated and improved on an
ongoing basis" (National Nursing Staff Development Organization, 1995).

**258**

## COMPETENCE VERSUS COMPETENCY

In today's complex healthcare setting, possession of credentials established through licensing and knowledge-based testing is an inadequate means of measuring competence. Ideal job performance in nursing is no longer task oriented but outcome oriented. A task-oriented nurse may provide safe care by following physicians' orders and organizational policies and by using technical skills. An outcome-oriented nurse will also use critical thinking and interpersonal skills to affect the progress of the patient and thus produce a better outcome. A better outcome may be, for example, a decreased length of stay or increased customer satisfaction. Interpersonal skills can be used to improve communication with physicians, peers, patients, and families. Critical thinking skills include anticipating problems, taking preventive action, and troubleshooting problems to move the patient positively along the pathway of the medical plan of care. This expanded interpretation of competence is embodied in the term *competency.*

*Competency* is defined as the integration of knowledge and technical, interpersonal, and critical thinking skills applied to patient care in a designated role and work setting, according to predetermined standards of practice.

Fig. 9-1 represents the dynamic nature of competency, showing the interaction of the elements of competency within a specific context. Competency, and therefore performance, is critically dependent on the work context, both at the unit and organizational level (del Bueno, 1990).

## INFLUENCING COMPETENCY

What happens when a nurse is "floated" out of his or her usual work setting? Safe practice of skills that are commonly performed in the usual work setting is now at risk. Why? Because the integration of all the elements of competency dynamics is disrupted, and the standard of performance will deteriorate until the elements are once more integrated. Knowledge about location of supplies, physicians'

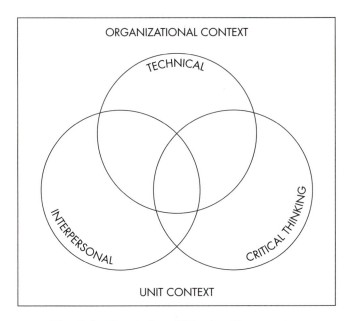

**Fig. 9-1** Dynamics of Nursing Competency.

preferences, protocols, routines, standards of practice, personalities, roles, and other factors influence this disruption. For the same reasons, safe practice of infrequently performed skills in any work setting jeopardizes competency and places the patient at risk.

Competency lies on a continuum (Fig. 9-2) influenced by the elements just described, but above all it is influenced by experience (Benner, 1984). Once achieved, competency must be maintained by practice. To borrow a couple of well-worn phrases: "Use it or lose it" and "Practice makes perfect." Now, let's take a closer look at Fig. 9-2.

## THE CONTINUUM OF COMPETENCY

A competent nurse is one whose performance integrates the dynamic elements of competency into patient care based on predetermined standards. Standards of practice are usually minimum requirements, providing guidelines for

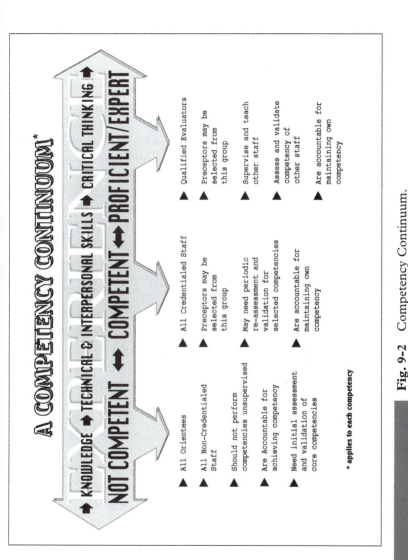

**Fig. 9-2**   Competency Continuum.

safe patient care in a given situation. An inexperienced nurse becomes competent when the rules and routines have been learned and practiced within the context of the work setting and performance is based on standards of practice. When continued experience is combined with the dynamic elements of competency, first proficient performance will occur and later expert performance will result, virtually in direct proportion to the degree of experience (Benner, 1984). Therefore it stands to reason that frequency of performance is critical to the development and maintenance of competency. It is important to remember that movement along the competency continuum—from not competent to competent, from proficient to expert—is specific for each skill. The absence of practice in a particular skill moves previously competent/expert performance back down the continuum, in almost direct proportion to frequency. It is important to identify clearly which nurses can be categorized in the three groups: (1) not competent, (2) competent, and (3) proficient/expert.

The *not-competent group* includes all new orientees, that is, new hires and transfers from other work settings. (Remember, context is critical to competency.) Even very experienced nurses who are new to a work setting may temporarily revert to the not-competent level of performance until the new rules are learned and the elements of competency dynamics can be reintegrated into practice.

The not-competent group also includes staff who have never demonstrated competency in a particular skill—either a new skill or an infrequently performed one. All staff cannot maintain competency for infrequently performed skills. In current "competency" jargon, these staff are not yet *credentialed.*

The not-competent group (1) should not perform care unsupervised, (2) needs initial assessment and validation of core (all frequently performed) skills, and (3) is accountable for achieving competency within a specified time frame.

The competent group includes all staff who are credentialed; that is, they have demonstrated competency on the job or in a simulated situation, or competency has been demonstrated by exception or default. Staff in this group would have demonstrated competency in core skills during orientation and in infrequently performed skills on an individual as-needed basis. *Competency by default* or *by exception* means that a unit-based organizational quality improvement program failed to reveal problems with a particular skill. If there are no problems, there is nothing to fix! The result is assessment and validation of competency by exception or default.

The *competent group:* (1) may need periodic assessment and validation of selected skills, and (2) is accountable for maintaining competency. Preceptors may be selected from the competent group. There is evidence to support the fact that the competent though relatively inexperienced nurse performs the preceptor role well with novice orientees because such a nurse is more likely (than a more experienced nurse) to be aware of orientees' needs (Benner, 1984).

The proficient/expert group is the one from which preceptors and qualified evaluators should be selected. This group (1) supervises and teaches other staff, (2) assesses and validates competency of other staff (qualified evaluators), and (3) is accountable for maintaining its level of competency. Remember: Competency is skill-selective; an expert in one skill may be at the not-competent level in another.

## A PLAN FOR COMPETENCY

Since competency is specific to context, any plan to ensure a competent staff must be unit based. The overall plan is the same, regardless of work setting. The plan must include methods to (1) assess and validate competency of all staff according to the job description and any special role requirements, (2) reveal the absence of competency, (3) resolve the absence of competency, and (4) support the development of competency for new skills. There are three phases in a holistic plan to assess and validate competency. In phase 1 the competency of all new hires is established during the orientation program. In phase 2 the maintenance of competency in the incumbent staff is monitored and deficiencies are

---

## ☀ Management Spotlight

*BACK UP OTHERS WHO NEED HELP*

(The Best Way to Put a Safety Net Under the Team's Performance)

- Back each other up
- Need a good feel for teammate's roles (see the big picture)
- Broaden skills
- Attitude of helpfulness

From Pritchett, P. (1997). *The team member handbook for teamwork.* Dallas: Pritchett & Associates.

---

resolved. In phase 3 competency in new skills and low-frequency skills is established. These three phases are presented in Fig. 9-3.

### Phase 1

Phase 1 assesses and validates acceptable performance of core skills (i.e., the commonly performed skills of the job) by all orientees, including transfers from other work settings within the organization. This phase is the foundation of the plan. The key to success of phase 1 is the establishment of a competency-based orientation program that is managed by trained, committed preceptors and implemented during the orientation period of the new job. Identification of core skills by the unit-based staff is also a key requirement. Tools are supplied and explained, with step-by-step instructions on page 264.

### Phase 2

Phase 2 assesses and validates continuous, consistent, and acceptable performance of core skills of the incumbent staff. The key to the success of this phase is the development of a unit-based quality improvement (QI) program that will track significant indicators of problems. This program should

**Fig. 9-3**  Unit-Based Competency Assessment and Validation Plan.
(Courtesy Heartland Regional Medical Center, St. Joseph, MO.)

UNIT-BASED COMPETENCY ASSESSMENT and VALIDATION PLAN

**PHASE 1**
**INITIAL ASSESSMENT OF COMPETENCY**

DEFINITION:

Acceptable performance of the core competencies of the job.

Involves establishing a competency-based orientation program

WHEN ASSESSED?
☺ During orientation to the new job

METHODS & TOOLS

Standards of Practice

Identification of core competencies

Competency Checklist for each core competency

Qualified Evaluators (Preceptors)

**PHASE 2**
**MAINTENANCE OF COMPETENCY**

DEFINITION:

Continuous, consistent, acceptable performance of core competencies.

Involves establishing
• a unit-based QI program
• a communication system

WHEN ASSESSED?
☺ By exception whenever performance does not meet standards of practice

METHODS & TOOLS

Practice Standards

Incident reports

Concern/Communication Forms *from physicians/patients/families and staff*

QI Indicators/Monitors

**PHASE 3**
**CONTINUOUS DEVELOPMENT OF COMPETENCY**

DEFINITION:

Performance development for new or low-frequency competencies.

Involves:
• periodic evaluation of low-frequency competencies
• "just-in-time" education and evaluation for new competencies

WHEN ASSESSED?
☺ When problems are identified for low-frequency competencies.
☺ When new competencies are generated.

METHODS & TOOLS

Identification of low-frequency competencies & development of competency checklists.

Periodic evaluation of low-frequency competencies.

"just-in-time" education for new procedures, or new equipment, etc.

Development of new competency checklists

**Competency-Based Education**

include monitoring of selected standards of practice and a communication system for customer complaints and staff concerns. It should be flexible in response to resulting data. If monitoring an indicator reveals no problem over a reasonable period, then another indicator should be monitored. It is assumed that a QI program exists at the organizational level to track problems such as infection rates, complications, returns to a more intensive level of care, mortality, incident reports, and customer complaints to provide a comprehensive data bank. This approach is assessment and validation of competency by exception or by default. If no problems are identified, there is nothing to fix!

Herding staff through annual "skill fairs," which has become a new tradition in competency management, is a waste of time and resources. It solves no problems but certainly creates some, not least of which is anger and resentment among staff members who are required to demonstrate skills that they frequently perform competently on the job. Problems that are identified may apply only to individual staff members or to the entire staff. Additionally, careful analysis of the problems is necessary to identify the cause. Education is not the universal solution. Experience reveals that noncompliance with policies and protocols is the more common cause. Problem solving by the staff is the solution to noncompliance. When learning needs are identified, each one should be addressed independently in terms of the best method to meet the need and solve the problem. Collaboration with an educator is recommended.

**Phase 3**

Phase 3 takes care of the competency development for new and low-frequency skills. New skills are generated by changes in procedure or policy or by new equipment or technology. The key to success for establishing competency in new skills is *just-in-time education,* followed by identification of a standard of practice indicator(s) and then monitoring of the new skill for a reasonable period. If no problem is identified, there is nothing to fix. Again, competency assessment and validation are done by default. Just-in-time education means providing adequate training sessions for all staff who will be required to perform the skill, including both theory and practice, and strategically timing the education for the period immediately before implementation of the new skill.

### Low-Frequency Skills

Low-frequency skills require a different approach. How does a nurse achieve and maintain competency of skills that are performed infrequently—half-yearly, yearly, or even less frequently? The solution is to develop a core group of credentialed staff, small enough to allow maintenance of competency by practice, yet large enough to be available whenever that skill is needed. When the need for that skill arises, a credentialed staff member may either supervise a noncredentialed member who is performing the skill or perform the skill himself or herself. This core of credentialed staff should be self-regulating and accountable for competent performance of the skill in question. Periodic education regarding this skill and assessment and validation of performance may be necessary. Developing a small core group of credentialed staff for each high-risk, low-frequency skill is a more cost-effective solution than dealing with the consequences of a negative outcome of incompetent performance.

### IMPLEMENTING THE PLAN
### Step 1

Step 1 is to choose a group of experienced staff, preferably those who have had some experience orienting new hires, to identify the unit-based skills. Use the *Unit-Based Skills Matrix Tool* (Fig. 9-4) to rate the frequency and risk for all the skills. This tool is self-explanatory and offers some plausible examples. Then complete the category label. It is debatable whether a skill that is performed approximately once per month is high frequency or low frequency. It depends on how many staff are involved. A small number of staff may be able to perform the skill sufficiently often to maintain competency. If that is the case, rate it as a core skill (high frequency). All competencies that are rated as high frequency are the core skills. These are the skills that make up the foundation of the competency-based orientation program. These core skills must be performed competently before the end of orientation. The low-frequency skills are those that fall under phase 3 of the unit-based plan (see Fig. 9-4).

## Step 2

Step 2 involves writing the competency checklists. A competency checklist is not the same as a traditional skills checklist.

---

**UNIT-BASED SKILLS MATRIX**

UNIT:_____
DATE:_____

List below the nursing skills performed in your unit with the corresponding *frequency and risk* rating.

Frequency refers to the number of times performed, based on a yearly average, and should be classified under D, W, M, or Y, (*daily, weekly, monthly, yearly*). A frequency of D or W (*daily or weekly*) means high frequency (H); a frequency of M or Y (*monthly or yearly*) means low frequency (L).

Risk means that if the procedure or skill is not done, or not done correctly, the patient and/or organization will be placed in jeopardy. Risk should be classified as High or Moderate (H or M).

Category Label is the combination of frequency and risk. A high-frequency, moderate-risk skill will have a category label of H/M. A low-frequency, high-risk skill will have the category label L/H.

➢ For each skill, place a check mark in the appropriate column for Frequency and Risk; then complete the Category Label

| *UNIT-BASED SKILLS* | FREQUENCY | | | | RISK | | CATEGORY LABEL |
|---|---|---|---|---|---|---|---|
| | D | W | M | Y | H | M | |
| Intravenous Therapy | ✓ | | | | ✓ | | H/H |
| Patient Transfer | ✓ | | | | | ✓ | H/M |
| Patient Admission | ✓ | | | | | ✓ | H/M |
| Epidural Analgesia | | ✓ | | | ✓ | | L/H |
| Cardiac Monitoring | ✓ | | | | ✓ | | H/H |
| Management of a Central Venous Catheter | | ✓ | | | ✓ | | H/H |
| Insertion of a Central Venous Catheter | | | | ✓ | ✓ | | L/H |
| Communication with the Physician | ✓ | | | | ✓ | | H/H |
| Pleural Under-Water-Seal Drain | | | ✓ | | ✓ | | L/H |
| Etc. | | | | | | | |
| | | | | | | | |
| | | | | | | | |
| | | | | | | | |

**Fig. 9-4**  Unit-Based Skills Matrix.

(Courtesy Heartland Regional Medical Center, St. Joseph, MO.)

Neither is it a step-by-step list of tasks to be performed, such as a protocol or procedure might appear. A competency checklist includes not only the technical skills but also the knowledge and critical thinking skills involved in the competent performance of a particular skill. Additionally, the competency checklist contains only the criteria that are critical to competent performance (i.e., must be performed for effectiveness and/or patient safety) (Fig. 9-5). Each performance criterion on the checklist is described in terms that can be measured (objectively observed). Each criterion should

*Heartland Health System*

**COMPETENCY CHECKLIST**

NAME:_____UNIT:_____
　　　　　　　　Please Print

| Resuscitates using Basic Life Support (BLS) and the Automated External Defibrillator (AED) | COMPLETED | |
|---|---|---|
| PERFORMANCE CRITERIA | RATING SCALE | Date/ Evaluator's Initials |
| 1.  Explains the rationale for early defibrillation. | I  S  A  M  D | |
| 2.  Follows policy to implement Code Blue response. | I  S  A  M  D | |
| 3.  Performs BLS until AED available. | I  S  A  M  D | |
| 4.  Places QUICK COMBO electrodes as soon as AED available. | I  S  A  M  D | |
| 5.  Pushes ANALYZE, standing clear of patient. | I  S  A  M  D | |
| 6.  Pushes CHARGE, if shock advised. | I  S  A  M  D | |
| 7.  Pushes SHOCK buttons simultaneously when joules available, ensuring all personnel stand clear of patient. | I  S  A  M  D | |
| 8.  Repeats steps 5 through 7 if advised, giving a total of 3 shocks, using 200, 200-300 & 360 J for each successive shock, with no pulse check in between. | I  S  A  M  D | |
| 9.  Performs pulse check after 3 shocks or if change in rhythm is observed. | I  S  A  M  D | |
| 10. If no pulse, continues BLS for 1 minute then repeats steps 5 through 10, using 360 J for shock # 4 and thereafter. | I  S  A  M  D | |
| 11. Takes action based on messages on AED monitor screen. | I  S  A  M  D | |
| 12. Explains electrical safety precautions. | I  S  A  M  D | |

*Successful completion requires a rating of "I" or "S". Ratings less than "I" or "S" require completion of an Education Action Plan.*

EVALUATOR'S NAME_____SIGNATURE_____
　　　　　　　　　　Please Print

COMMENTS:

**Fig. 9-5**　Competency Checklist.
(Courtesy Heartland Regional Medical Center, St. Joseph, MO.)

Competency-Based Education

include only one behavior (del Bueno, 1995). Use existing publications (e.g., Lohrman & Kinkade, 1992) that include competency checklists; these can be modified and individualized to suit your work setting.

The amount of detail written into each criterion statement is a matter of choice. Ideally, the evaluator of performance is proficient or expert at the skill; therefore that person will know the details, and it will not be necessary to write them all on the checklist. For example, refer to statements 1, 2, 4, and 11 listed in Fig. 9-5. The evaluator should know the rationale for early defibrillation; the code blue policy; how, where, and when to place the electrodes; and what actions to take based on data obtained during the procedure. These statements are evaluating the knowledge and critical thinking component of the skill. However, the competency checklist can also be a learning tool for the staff being evaluated. A little extra detail written into each statement is helpful in this situation, especially when a new skill is involved (as in this case).

Refer to the Rating Scale on the checklist. Logically, one is either competent or not competent in an area; one cannot be partly competent. However, evaluators, who are staff themselves (albeit expert), often find it difficult to categorize their peers as not competent. Experience has shown that evaluators find it easier to rate their peers according to a scale (Fig. 9-6). This rating can assist in identifying learning needs when staff do not meet the ideal rating. Nervousness caused by the testing nature of the evaluation and the mere fact of being watched interferes with competent performance. Some cueing by the evaluator may be necessary to overcome the inherent problems of performing under scrutiny in these circumstances. Using a rating scale allows for a definition of safe and accurate performance with verbal cueing. However, if performance is accurate only if verbal and/or physical direction must be given, then a rating of "A" will not support competent performance. When performance of any criterion has been rated less than "I" or "S," it is easier to see whether the staff member's learning needs require an education plan (Fig. 9-7) or can be met relatively easily by a quick correction and review,

## Performance Evaluation Tool

| Rating Scale Label | Standard for Performance | Quality of Performance | Assistance |
|---|---|---|---|
| Independent (I) | Safe, accurate | Is efficient, competent, coordinated, confident; performs within an expedient time period | Without supportive cues |
| Supervised (S) | Safe, accurate | Is competent, coordinated, and confident; shows some expenditure of excess energy; performs within a reasonable time period | Occasional supportive cues |
| Assisted (A) | Safe, accurate | Is skillful in most parts of behavior; shows inefficiency and a degree of incoordination; expends excess energy; performs within a delayed time period | Frequent verbal and occasional physical directive cues in addition to supportive ones |
| Marginal (M) | Safe but not alone, performing at risk, not always accurate | Is unskilled, inefficient; shows considerable expenditure of excess energy and lack of coordination; performs within a prolonged time period | Continuous verbal and frequent physical cues |
| Dependent (D) | Unsafe, inability to demonstrate behavior | Is unable to demonstrate procedure/behavior; lacks confidence, coordination, and efficiency | Continuous verbal and physical cues |
| Not Applicable (N) | Currently unable to perform procedure/behavior due to unavailability of opportunity or approved delay in seeking opportunity. | | |

**Fig. 9-6**   Performance Evaluation Tool. For successful completion of this competency, performance must be rated at not less than the "S" (Supervised) Level. A rating below "S" requires an Education Action Plan.

Modified from Bondy K. N. (1983). Criterion-referenced definitions for rating scales in clinical evaluation. *J Hursing Education*, 22(9): 376-382.

**Fig. 9-7** Education Action Plan. (Courtesy Heartland Regional Medical Center, St. Joseph, MO.)

*Heartland Health System*

EDUCATION ACTION PLAN

NAME: _____ TITLE: _____ UNIT: _____

(Please Print)

PROBLEM/ LEARNING NEED:

| PLAN | | | | | |
|---|---|---|---|---|---|
| Objectives | Strategies/ Activities | Evaluation Methods | Date Commenced | Target Date | Date Completed |
| | | | | | |
| | | | | | |

COMMENTS: _____

SIGNATURES: _____ _____ Date: _____

Staff Member     Manager

1 COPY - STAFF MEMBER     1 COPY - MANAGER

followed by a repeat assessment of the criteria statements involved. Any learning needs that are not being met at the time of the assessment should be included in an education plan, with the goal being demonstration of competent performance. If the rating scale is used, it is essential that all evaluators "buy into" its value and become familiar with the application of the criteria of the scale through practice sessions.

The rating scale is particularly valuable during competency-based orientation. Preceptors can clearly document weak and strong areas to guide learning experiences during orientation and to document competent performance of all required core skills and readiness to terminate the orientation period. Additionally, this type of rating provides documentation of unsatisfactory performance for orientees and incumbent staff to support disciplinary action after reasonable efforts have been made to meet learning needs.

Together, these tools—the unit-based skills checklist, the competency (performance) checklist, the rating scale, and the education plan—provide the means to document successful and unsuccessful performance of orientees and incumbent staff and the efforts at resolution of performance problems.

## Step 3

Use the unit-based skills checklist to select the skills that are high frequency in your work setting, and place the corresponding competency checklists in an orientation manual. Then, when a new orientee is hired, select the appropriate skills to be assessed and validated during orientation, depending on the experience of the orientee. A new RN graduate may need assessment and validation of the more simple skills. A more experienced orientee will probably not need to be assessed on all core skills. Keep the orientation manual easily accessible so staff can review and update the criteria in the checklists as necessary. As new high-frequency skills are required by policy and procedure changes, develop the competency checklists and add them to the manual. Select the preceptors who will be the key players in the competency-based

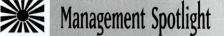 **Management Spotlight**

*HELP NEW TEAMMATES MAKE ENTRY*

- When a newcomer fails to make it in the team, it is often because the team failed the person.
- It is to the team's advantage to support them and get them settled ASAP.

From Pritchett, P. (1997). *The team member handbook for teamwork.* Dallas: Pritchett.

orientation program, and provide them with adequate support and education to perform their role and use the tools. This is phase 1 of the competency assessment and validation plan.

Now select the skills that are low frequency. Place the corresponding competency checklists in another easily available manual. Update the manual as new low-frequency skills are required and as the checklists are developed (described in phase 3 of the competency assessment and validation plan).

**Step 4**

Step 4 deals with phase 2 of the plan. A performance problem is identified through the QI program, and it involves a large number of the staff. After careful analysis of the problem, a decision is made to provide education and then to assess and validate competency. These steps need to be followed:

1. Plan the educational strategy to meet the specific learning needs of the staff, and estimate the time required to complete it.
2. Plan the method that will be used to assess and validate competent performance (e.g., a simulated station or evaluation of actual on-the-job performance). Estimate the time required to complete it.
3. Set a realistic time line.

4. Select the qualified evaluators according to the recommended criteria (Fig. 9-8).

5. Develop the evaluation tool, usually a competency (performance) checklist (Box 9-1). Include in it all the knowledge and critical thinking components of the skill in question, as well as in the critical performance steps. Avoid written tests, which measure knowledge only. Critical knowledge should be included on the checklist to be used during the performance assessment.

6. Provide all staff with information about the assessment and validation method, the tool to be used, and the time frame for completion. Clarify their accountability for achieving competency and the consequences of unsuccessful performance.

7. Set up practice stations for qualified evaluators. Qualified evaluators should develop a detailed worksheet corresponding to the criteria on the checklist to ensure that everyone has the same expectations and standards for meeting each criterion. Then they should check each other's criteria off against the standards established. The station can be improved or modified at this stage. Estimate the time it will take to assess each person.

8. Set up practice stations for staff to attend on a voluntary basis. This approach will promote accountability and decrease anxiety.

9. Schedule staff for specific times to be assessed. This method will reduce the time taken for assessment to a minimum and will facilitate scheduling of staff and evaluators. Assessment should always be carried out on an individualized basis. Provide privacy and a calm, quiet environment.

10. Ensure documentation of the whole process, including a roster of attendance.

11. Meet with evaluators for debriefing, and review any evidence of unsuccessful performance. Develop an education plan, and meet with the staff involved to implement the plan.

12. Set up a QI monitor for the skill in question to validate resolution of the problem.

**Heartland Regional Medical Center**

**Policy No. MS. 159**

**COMPETENCY ASSESSMENT AND VALIDATION**

**Chairperson, Management Council** **DATE**

### Defining Statement

Competency is defined as the integration of knowledge, attitude, critical thinking, and interpersonal and practical skills applied to the care of the patient in a designated role and setting, which conforms to pre-determined standards to ensure safe practice.

### Policy Statement

All professional staff will demonstrate and maintain competency according to their scope of practice and job description.

Competency is assessed according to standards of care, and Heartland Hospital policies and procedures.

Unsuccessful completion of competency assessment will require an education plan with successful completion in 3 months. Unsuccessful completion of an education plan will result in participant being unable to perform those functions until reassessment.

Competency is reviewed at regular intervals based on the following:

- findings from quality improvement monitoring
- mandatory requirements of Acute Care Nursing Division; e.g., BLS, blood transfusion, etc.
- new and/or changing technology
- new and/or changing knowledge related to research-based practice
- care delivery changes
- new or revised nursing policies and procedures
- identified learning needs of the staff

Plans for each competency to be assessed (e.g., care of the patient requiring chest tubes, care of the patient requiring hyperalimentation, etc.) will include the following:

- identified source of learning need or purpose (Why are you doing this? e.g., high risk - low volume, QI, etc.)
- target staff
- objectives
- methods/evaluation tools
- time frame
- designated qualified evaluators
- reference sources for content of evaluation tools
- defined criteria for successful completion

**Fig. 9-8, *A*** Competency Assessment and Validation.

(Courtesy Heartland Regional Medical Center, St. Joseph, MO.)

Qualified evaluators who possess the experience, education, clinical knowledge, and skills appropriate to the specific area will assess and validate competency. Criteria for qualified evaluators:

1. Knowledgeable about specific competency
2. Recognized by their peers as proficient (as described by Benner) in the specific competency
3. One year clinical experience related to specific competency
4. Willingness to participate
5. No disciplinary action in progress
6. Professional commitment: e.g., actively involved in professional organization, show concern for QI in practice.
7. Certification by a nationally recognized organization in their specialty area
8. Experience in competency assessment: e.g., preceptor, ACLS/BLS/PALS/NALS instructor, clinical/patient instructor
9. Involvement in educational process in clinical area.

**NOTE:** #1 - 6 = mandatory requirement

The Education Department will be responsible for:

- advising on the competency assessment and validation process
- grading and scoring of competency assessment
- notification of results to Team Leader within three working days
- Development of an education plan with input from appropriate Team Leader within five working days.
- monitoring implementation of education plan during three month time frame
- documentation of competency results

The Team Leader will be responsible for:

- input in developing an education plan
- follow up and documentation with involved parties throughout the 3 months implementation of the education plan

**References:**

Benner, Patricia (1984). *From Novice to Expert,* Menlo Park, CA: Addison Wesley.

Joint Commission on Accreditation of Healthcare Organizations (JCAHO), (1994). 1995 *Accreditation manual for hospitals: Vol 1 Standards.* Oakbrook Terrace, Ill.: Author.

Joint Commission on Accreditation of Healthcare Organizations (JCAHO), (1993). Nursing competency assessment: *Regaining control of the Process.* Oakbrook Terrace, Ill.: Author.

Lohrman, J.M. & Kinkade, S.L. (1992). *Competency-based orientation for critical care nursing.* St. Louis: Mosby.

Robinson, S.M. & Barberis-Ryan, C. (1996). *Competency assessment: A systematic approach.* Nursing Management, 26(2), 40-44.

1/23/91
Revised 02/08/93
Revised 9/95
Revised 8/96

CREDENT.ADM

*Courtesy of Heartland Regional Medical Center, St. Joseph, MO*

**Fig. 9-8, *B*** Cont'd. Competency Assessment and Validation.

Competency-Based Education

---

**BOX 9-1**

## COMPETENCY/CREDENTIALING PLAN

**COMPETENCIES:** Manages Daily Crash-Cart Checks and Crash-Cart Exchange

### Needs Assessment
- This is a high-risk, medium-frequency competency for most nurses in the critical care department—low frequency for some.
- Opportunities need to be made available for practice.
- 100% compliance is required by JCAHO on this type of activity.
- QI process revealed noncompliance.

### Target Staff
All RNs who work in the critical care department and who are no longer in orientation.

### Program Objectives
To provide an opportunity for knowledge and skill update through guided self-study and practice in a simulated situation
To assess learning needs
To validate competency and promote 100% compliance with code-cart checks

### Methods/Strategies
1. Provide material for self-study and copies of competency checklist
2. Provide teaching sessions on units with own crash-cart equipment at times appropriate for staff
3. Schedule staff periodically, in groups or individually, for validation of competency at simulated stations
4. Ensure adequate communication with staff re-credentialing plans; i.e., individual letters with instructions, fliers, material in self-study manuals; unit-based education representatives well informed and providing information at staff meeting

### Evaluation Tools/Methods
Competency stations with crash-cart, defibrillator/cardioverter to create a simulated situation for performance

Competency checklist to be successfully completed at the "S" level on Bondy's Rating Scale (*see attached competency checklist*)

May be evaluated only by a qualified evaluator, approved by the critical care education subcommittee

*Continued*

---

### BOX 9-1—Cont'd

**Criteria for Successful Completion of Competency**
A rating of "I" or "S" on all criteria on the competency checklist

**Time Frame for Completion**
All staff successfully completed by end of December 1996

**Qualified Evaluators: Names/Credentials**
David Loyd, RN; Experienced critical care and PACU nurse; experienced in teaching and evaluating performance at the bedside and in other settings; is in a leadership role in the department and is the education representative; ACLS trained; preceptor

Wayne Smither, RN; experienced critical care nurse; experienced in bedside teaching and performance evaluation; preceptor; ACLS Instructor

Vivien Jutsum, RN; critical care educator; ACLS coordinator and instructor; experienced in teaching and evaluation at the bedside and in simulated situations

Mary Herring, RN; experienced critical care nurse; preceptor; ACLS trained

Margaret Wallace, RN; experienced critical care nurse; preceptor; ACLS trained

**References**
American Association of Critical Care Nurses (AACN), 1993. *AACN Procedure Manual for Critical Care,* 3rd. ed. Philadelphia: Saunders.

American Heart Association, 1994. *Textbook of Advanced Cardiac Life Support.* Dallas: Author.

Heartland Health System policies.

---

Courtesy Heartland Regional Medical Center, St. Joseph, MO.

---

## DOCUMENTATION OF COMPETENCY ASSESSMENT AND VALIDATION

It is not necessary to keep a completed competency checklist for each person for each skill assessed. Develop a summary documentation for persons who successfully achieve competency, or include each person's achievement in the computerized education recordkeeping system. All education plans should be filed in a personnel record when completed. Documentation of resolution of performance problems is essential. This documentation can be written in stages as the steps listed in the preceding section are followed. This approach will help to promote development of a sound plan based on rational analysis of the problem.

## CONCLUSION

Competency is not a checklist of tasks or skills. It is performance rated against the standards by qualified evaluators. Competency is performance that improves patient care outcomes. The competency assessment plan must focus on performance that is assessed against predetermined standards of practice that are relevant to the work setting. Performance is best assessed on the job; the next best method is a setting that simulates on-the-job performance. Development of a QI program and a competency-based orientation program is the foundation for the plan. Together, these two components establish a baseline of documented competency and a means of monitoring the development of problems. Special consideration must be given to the development and maintenance of competency for low-frequency skills and new skills. The value of developing preceptors and qualified evaluators as the "keepers" and standard setters of competency should not be underestimated. Finally, documentation of competency assessment and validation and resolution of performance problems are invaluable in validating unit-based performance achievements and standards of practice that improve outcomes of care.

## BIBLIOGRAPHY

Benner, P. (1984). *From novice to expert.* Menlo Park, CA: Addison-Wesley.

Bondy, K. N. (1983). Criterion-referenced definitions for rating scales in clinical evaluation. *Journal of Nursing Education, 22* (9), 376-382.

del Bueno, D. (1990). Evaluation: Myths, mystiques and obsessions. *Nursing Administration, 20* (11), 4-7.

del Bueno, D. (1995, October). *Competency development and evaluation do's and don'ts.* Paper presented at a symposium conducted at Kansas University Medical Center, Kansas City, KS.

Lohrman, J. M., & Kinkade, S. L. (1992). *Competency-based orientation for critical care nursing.* St. Louis: Mosby.

National Nursing Staff Development Organization (NNSDO). (1995). *Blueprint for competence: The University of Minnesota model.* (Ed., B. P. Puetz). Pensacola, FL: Author.

Robinson, S. M., & Barberis-Ryan, C. (1995). Competency assessment: A systematic approach. *Nursing Management, 26* (2), 40-44.

# Appendices
# Sample
# Management
# Tools

# Appendix A

# Unit Performance Improvement Plan

**MEDICAL CENTER—Patient Care Services Division**

## QUALITY IMPROVEMENT PLAN—MEDICAL/ SURGICAL UNITS

Effective Date: 1/97

---

Director, Medical/Surgical Units

**Purpose**
To provide a continuous monitoring system that supports quality of care for medical and surgical patients. The medical/surgical service supports the philosophy of the Medical Center, in the provision of quality services to all patients, with special attention to high-risk, high-frequency, or problem-prone areas.

**Responsibility**
The Vice President of Patient Care Services is ultimately responsible for the quality/performance improvement for Patient Care Services. The Director of Medical/Surgical, is responsible for the unit specific activities of medical and surgical floors. Major aspects of care will be monitored by the staff. Data analysis, submission of reports, and corrective action are the responsibility of the Director.

**Scope of Care**
The medical unit is a 37-bed unit providing acute, comprehensive nursing care for adult medical/surgical patients on a 24 hour per

Page 1

285

day, seven days per week basis. Types of medical patients admitted to the unit may include, but are not limited to: general, neurovascular, cardiac, pulmonary, and other chronic and infectious diseases.

In addition to general medicine, the medical unit specializes in the management of the patient with diabetes. The medical unit also frequently treats the overflow surgical population. The surgical unit is a 26-bed unit providing acute, comprehensive care for adult med/surg patients with primarily various interventions requiring general, orthopedic, urology, and neurovascular surgery. On occasion, the surgical unit treats the overflow medical population. Staff are cross-trained to function in either area when the fluctuation of staffing needs arise.

Nursing care is delivered within a Partners In Care conceptual framework. Generally, under the direction of a charge nurse, patients are assigned a team consisting of a registered nurse (RN) paired with either licensed or unlicensed assistive personnel. Nurse to patient ratios are established within the framework; however, acuity levels determined by *Medicus* and/or clinical judgements, may warrant nurse to patient ratios to be modified.

The licensed practical nurse (LPN) is formulated within the conceptual model as a Nursing Assistant, yet her duties and scope of practice remain the same. It is generally best to assign the LPN with the charge nurse, since her scope of practice allows her to be of greater assistance to the RN.

The psychosocial and spiritual needs of patients and their families are identified and supported by all staff, with the assistance of the continuing care discharge planning nurse, social worker, and pastoral care. Education is also an important service rendered to our patients and their families. Documentation of such care and treatment is maintained per hospital and unit policy.

Families are included as an integral part of the patient's plan of care. Family members receive instruction from staff members in necessary post discharge care requirements. These instructions frequently include urinary catheter care, venous access devices, anticoagulant therapy, enteral and total parental nutrition, oxygen delivery, telemetry monitoring, wound management, and home pain management. In addition, education related to diabetes management is also provided.

All patients are to be protected against potential complications related to care and treatments received on this unit. Protection is maximized through ongoing patient monitoring, and the application of safety devices, such as infusion pumps, side rails, restraints, and warning labels and signs. In addition, universal precautions, which include good handwashing skills, are also practiced.

**Performance Indicators To Be Monitored**
High-volume, high-risk, or problem-prone performance indicators will have priority for monitoring and evaluation on the medical/surgical service.

A. Sentinel Events
   1. Medication variances/Adverse drug reactions (ADRs)
   2. Patient falls
   3. Patient satisfaction scores
B. Concurrent Monthly Monitoring
   1. Documentation
   2. Infected vascular access devices
   3. Response time call lights
   4. Pain management
   5. Heparin therapy
   6. Nosocomial infections
C. Personnel Evaluation
   1. Job description
   2. Attitude
   3. Knowledge and skills
   4. Outputs (productivity; cost-effective practices; quality, customer-focused care)
   5. Accountability
   6. Interpersonal relationships (with co-workers and physicians)

Page 3

Sample Management Tools

# Appendix B

# Unit Vision

**MEDICAL CENTER—Patient Care Services Division**

---

## UNIT VISION—MEDICAL

Effective Date: 7/96

---

Director, Medical Unit

**Organizational Mission**
- To become a regional medical center
- To provide services through customer oriented care—our customers and *patients, visitors, physicians, volunteers,* and *fellow employees*
- To participate as partners with our Medical Staff
- To demonstrate continuous quality improvement programs
- To be fiscally sound
- To create an environment for employees that invites *teamwork, success,* and *pride*
- To create an atmosphere of open communications with the community

**UNIT VISION**
**Mission/Purpose**
To provide medical services through customer-oriented care. We involve patients and families in all aspects of care during and after their hospitalization. We put the patients' and families' needs first.

**Unit Standards:**
- To work collaboratively with others.
- To be accountable for the outcomes on our unit.
- To have an open environment that fosters creativity and innovation.

Page 1

---

288

**Key Values**
Each staff member will be self-confident, self-motivated, and self-managed.

Each staff member demonstrates professional pride through interpersonal interactions, cleanliness of the unit, and positive outcomes from patient care.

Each staff member contributes to the unity of purpose/concern as it relates to the medical team.

**Nursing Process**
- The nursing process emphasizes quality and individualized patient care.
- The nursing process assists staff to achieve more consistent and higher quality of care.
- Through the collaborative efforts of the nurse and patient, a clear practical care plan is developed and utilized to achieve a positive outcome.

**Unit Image**
- The staff are motivated and inspire confidence.
- The staff demonstrate high standards and high level of professionalism.
- Each other's opinions are valued and each give timely feedback and strive to keep each other informed.
- Others recognize the medical unit for its vast diversity of chronic and acute disease processes; however, the expertise can be found in the care of the patient with diabetes.
- Staff treat each other with courtesy, consideration, and professional respect.

**Performance Improvement Initiatives**
***Personnel Evaluations.*** In addition to the individual job description, employees are also evaluated on *attitude, knowledge, and skills outputs* (productivity, cost-effective practices, and quality patient care); *accountability;* and *interpersonal relationships* (with co-workers and physicians).

***Quality Improvement Initiatives.*** To provide a continuous monitoring system that supports quality of care for medical/surgical patients. The medical unit supports the philosophy of (name of institution) in the provision of quality, customer-oriented services to all patients, with special attention to the high-risk, high-frequency, or problem-prone areas. (See Medical Unit QI Plan.)

# Appendix C

# Interview Selection Tools

**GENERIC**

---

## INTERVIEWS

**Position:** _____   **Date:** _____

**Name:**   **Credentials:**

| *Questions* | *Comments* |
| --- | --- |

1. What is your knowledge base regarding workload management/acuity systems?
2. Describe your experiences in hiring and terminating employees.
3. Describe your experiences with the budget process.
4. Describe some situations in which you have considered yourself flexible.
5. Describe your experiences with budget control (i.e., orientation costs, patient acuity, and utilization of resources)
6. Describe previously developed policies, teaching tools, or checklists.
7. How have you handled stressful situations in the past?
8. Describe your style of leadership/management.

Page 1

---

## INTERVIEWS

Position: _____    Date: _____

Name:                                Credentials:

| Questions | Comments |
|---|---|
| 9. If selected, what do you feel you could bring to this position? | |
| 10. Describe your interactive skills in dealing with staff and physicians. | |
| 11. What do you think are the most important characteristics of an effective nursing manager? | |
| 12. How would you describe the ideal boss? | |
| 13. How would you handle a situation where you disagree with administrative policy or decision? | |
| 14. What are your strengths? | |
| 15. What are your weaknesses? | |
| 16. Describe your experiences with the application of progressive discipline. | |
| 17. Describe your experience with assuring that quality improvement standards established for the unit are met consistently for all patients. | |
| 18. Describe how you would provide for adequate replacement of human resources to assure consistency in scheduling and staffing levels required by patient volume and acuity. | |
| 19. a. Describe your experience with the planning and design of operational enhancements in areas of responsibility. | |
| b. What is your experience with benchmarking? | |

Page 2

Sample Management Tools

**NURSE MANAGER**

## M/S CONSOLIDATION SELECTION TOOL

**Nurse Manager:** _____ **Unit:** _____

Scale: 1-5
1 = Least Favorable
5 = Most Favorable

| Attributes | 1 | 2 | 3 | 4 | 5 | Comments |
|---|---|---|---|---|---|---|
| 1. Degree of Leadership Demonstrated: <br> a. Challenging Processes <br> b. Inspiring a Shared Vision <br> c. Enabling Others to Act <br> d. Modeling the Way | | | | | | |
| 2. Degree of Initiative Demonstrated | | | | | | |
| 3. Attitudes/Interpersonal Skills | | | | | | |
| 4. Physician Relationships | | | | | | |
| 5. Staff Relationships/ Interactions | | | | | | |
| 6. Demonstration of Flexibility | | | | | | |
| 7. Unique Characteristics, Qualifications for Clinical Position | | | | | | |
| 8. Identified Leadership Roles | | | | | | |
| 9. Education/ Certification/CE | | | | | | |
| 10. Latest MBD Score | | | | | | |
| 11. Total Years Service <br> Total Years NM Role | | | | | | |
| 13. Other | | | | | | |

Comments:

## STAFFING COORDINATOR/NURSING SUPERVISOR

# ADMINISTRATIVE SUPERVISOR/STAFFING COORDINATOR—SCORING TOOL

| Points | 1 | 2 | 3 | 4 | Points |
|---|---|---|---|---|---|
| Education level | <30 HR AD | <60 HR BS | BSN/BS | MS/MSN | |
| Inservices 1998 (Non mandatory includes critical care and hospital) | <10 HR | <15 HR | <20 HR | <30 HR | |
| Contact hrs/cont ed | <24 HR | <32 HR | <48 HR | <56 HR | |
| Previous experience | <6 YRS | <11 YRS | <16 YRS | <21 YRS | |
| Certifications | BCLS | INST. BCLS | NACLS | SPEC. CERT | |

Community activities
(Possible 1 pt each) _____

_____

Professional activities
(Possible 1 pt each) _____

_____

(Score each question 0-5)
Describe the protocol that would facilitate upward flow of information.

_____

_____

What is your knowledge base regarding workload management/ acuity systems?

_____

_____

Have you utilized workload management skills in your present unit?

_____

_____

_____

Page 1

# ADMINISTRATIVE SUPERVISOR/STAFFING COORDINATOR—SCORING TOOL

| Points | 1 | 2 | 3 | 4 | Points |
|---|---|---|---|---|---|

Do you have any staffing/workload management skills or experience?

Describe your experiences in hiring and terminating employees.

Briefly describe your view of scheduling as a recruitment and retention tool.

Describe some situations in which you have considered yourself flexible.

Describe your experiences with the budget process.

Describe your experiences with budget control (i.e., orientation costs patient acuity and utilization of resources)

Have you developed any checklists, teaching tools, or policies and procedures previously? (Describe some.)

Briefly describe your recent clinical experiences? Do you consider this important in your role as an administrative supervisor?

How have you handled stressful situations in the past?

## ADMINISTRATIVE SUPERVISOR/STAFFING COORDINATOR—SCORING TOOL

| Points | 1 | 2 | 3 | 4 | Points |
|---|---|---|---|---|---|

Describe your style of leadership/management.

_____

_____

What are your goals for the next three years?

_____

_____

Why are you seeking the staffing coordinator position?

_____

_____

What would your goals for staffing management include?

_____

_____

If selected, what do you feel you could bring to this position.

_____

_____

Describe your interactive skills in dealing with staff.

_____

_____

Comments:

_____

_____

Name_____ Date_____

Page 3

# Appendix D

# End of Shift Reports

CLINICAL SETTING/UNIT

---

## EASTERN NEW MEXICO MEDICAL CENTER
## END OF SHIFT REPORT— MEDICAL/ SURGICAL

Date: _____    Shift: _____    Unit: _____    Census: _____

| Admissions Room # | | Discharges Room # | | Surgeries Room # | | Emergency Procs Room # |
|---|---|---|---|---|---|---|
| | | | | | | |
| | | | | | | |
| | | | | | | |
| | | | | | | |
| | | | | | | Special Procedures |
| | | | | | | |
| | | | | | | |
| | | Outstanding Employee: | | | | |
| OBS Room # | | Why: | | | | |
| | | Outstanding M.D.: | | | | |
| | | Why: | | | | |

**Problems Related to:**

Bed Utilization _____

Physicians _____

Equipment/Supplies _____

Assignments/Co-Workers _____

Non-Productive Time _____

Other Departments _____

**Pace/Workload    Quiet    Steady    Busy    Very Busy**
_____

Courtesy of Eastern New Mexico Medical Center.

Page 1

296

# EASTERN NEW MEXICO MEDICAL CENTER END OF SHIFT REPORT— MEDICAL/ SURGICAL

**Report on Patients Who Develop (Include Room #)**

Decubitus Not Present on Admission _____

Decubitus Present On Admission That Worsens _____

Post-Op Respiratory Problems _____

Temp 101F or Greater_____

IV Phlebitis _____

IV Infiltrations _____

Post-Op Wound Infection _____

Blood Transfusion Errors _____

Number of Blood Transfusions _____

Complications with Epidurals or PCA Pumps _____

Hemorrhage _____

Colostomy Care _____

**Report Room Numbers for**

Code Blue _____        Falls/Injuries _____

Deaths _____        Med Occurrences _____

DNR _____

| Transfers (Room #s) |
| --- |
| Another Facility _____ |
| CCS _____ |
| Room Changes _____ |
| _____ |

Significant Events/Concerns/Comments _____

_____

_____

Signature(s): _____

Page 2

MULTIPLE UNITS/SUPERVISOR

# NURSING REPORT—STAFFING ADJUSTMENTS AND SHIFT ACTIVITY

Date: _____  Shift: _____  Nursing Supervisor: _____

| Unit | Staff Scheduled | C E N | Medicus | | Var | Adj | Unit | Staff Scheduled | C E N | Medicus | | Var | Adj |
|------|-----------------|-------|---------|--------|-----|-----|------|-----------------|-------|---------|--------|-----|-----|
| | | | | Actual | | | | | | | Actual | | |
| 2W | | | | | | | ER | | | | | | |
| 3S | | | | | | | ICU | | | | | | |
| TCU | | | | | | | L&D PP NURS | | | | | | |
| PEDS | | | | | | | 23 OBS | | | | | | |

Admissions:
Adm/transfer Delays (>30 mins):
Staffing Problems/Issues:
Director called/time:

Deaths/Codes:
Patient/Family Complaints:
Risk Mgmt Events/Employee Injuries:
Number of trips to: Pharmacy/Linen/Supply:
(time/unit)

**NURSING ACTIVITY TRACKING LOG**

# Nursing Activity Tracking Log

Month/Year                    Unit

| Date | Activity | Resource Person | Target Date | Follow-up/Comments |
|------|----------|-----------------|-------------|--------------------|
|      |          |                 |             |                    |
|      |          |                 |             |                    |
|      |          |                 |             |                    |
|      |          |                 |             |                    |
|      |          |                 |             |                    |
|      |          |                 |             |                    |
|      |          |                 |             |                    |
|      |          |                 |             |                    |
|      |          |                 |             |                    |
|      |          |                 |             |                    |
|      |          |                 |             |                    |
|      |          |                 |             |                    |
|      |          |                 |             |                    |
|      |          |                 |             |                    |
|      |          |                 |             |                    |
|      |          |                 |             |                    |
|      |          |                 |             |                    |
|      |          |                 |             |                    |
|      |          |                 |             |                    |
|      |          |                 |             |                    |
|      |          |                 |             |                    |
|      |          |                 |             |                    |
|      |          |                 |             |                    |
|      |          |                 |             |                    |
|      |          |                 |             |                    |
|      |          |                 |             |                    |
|      |          |                 |             |                    |
|      |          |                 |             |                    |
|      |          |                 |             |                    |
|      |          |                 |             |                    |
|      |          |                 |             |                    |
|      |          |                 |             |                    |

# Appendix E

# Orientation Summary Checklist

## MEDICAL/SURGICAL NURSE MANAGER

NAME: (Please print) _____

| Orientation Summary Checklist | | Completed |
|---|---|---|
| Learning Activities and Competencies | Target Date | Evaluator's Initials/Date |
| 1. Completes Hospital Orientation Program. | | |
| 2. Completes Nursing Orientation Program<br>  a. Medication Test<br>  b. Generic Skills Assessment Checklist<br>  c. Code Blue System<br>  d. Risk Management<br>  e. Quality Improvement Plan<br>  f. Pharmacy Overview<br>  g. IV Therapy Policy and Procedure<br>  h. LifeNet Organ Procurement | | |
| 3. a. Locates Equipment/Supplies/Resources<br>  b. Orients to Hospital Structure/Services (Scavenger Hunts) | | |
| 4. Completes Departmental Orientation Testing and Learning Needs Assessment:<br>  a. Medication Calculations<br>  b. Unit-based Skills Assessment Check-list | | |
| 5. Completes Computer Class:<br>  a. Order Communication<br>  b. BEDCOM | | |
| 6. Nurse-Call Communication System Competency. | | |

Page 1

300

# MEDICAL/SURGICAL NURSE MANAGER

NAME: (Please print) _____

| **Orientation Summary Checklist** | | **Completed** |
|---|---|---|
| **Learning Activities and Competencies** | **Target Date** | **Evaluator's Initials/Date** |
| 7. Completes 1 day with Unit Secretary. | | |
| 8. Orientation to Intercare—Marianne | | |
| 9. Orientation to Nurse Manager Role—<br>Ronnie F.—Budget/Staffing<br>Marianne W.—Leadership style,<br>record keeping, education<br>Anna P.—Leadership style, record<br>keeping, QE | | |
| 10. Blood Products Transfusion<br>Competency. | | |
| 11. Annual Mandatory Inservices<br>Fire and Safety/Hazardous Materials<br>Infection Control<br>BSI, Bloodborne Pathogens, TB &<br>Mask Fit<br>CPR | | |
| 12. Accucheck Competency (Quarterly)<br>—Kathy G. | | |
| 13. IV Therapy Competency/Midline—<br>Marianne (IV), Ronnie (Midline,<br>VADs, Mediport) | | |
| 14. Medication Cart Management | | |
| 15. Orientation to Budget Process—<br>Tom O. | | |
| 16. Staffing and Scheduling—<br>Marianne W., Ann G. | | |
| 17. Medicus—Ann G. | | |
| 18. Pain Management—Marty<br>a. Class/Self-Study<br>b. PCA Pump Bedside<br>Competency | | |

_____

Administrative Director Copy

Sample Management Tools

# ADDITIONAL LEARNING ACTIVITIES AND COMPETENCIES

NAME: (Please print) _____

| Orientation Summary Checklist | | Completed |
|---|---|---|
| **Learning Activities and Competencies** | **Target Date** | **Evaluator's Initials/Date** |
| 19. Care of the Patient receiving Epidural Analgesia | | |
| 20. Care of the patient with:<br>a. Long-term Venous Access Device —Joanne B.<br>b. Implantable port<br>c. Midline Catheter | | |
| 21. EKG Interpretation Course | | |
| 22. Infection Control—Jackie B. | | |
| 23. QM | | |
| 24. Quality Improvement—Sandy C. | | |
| 25. Risk Management—Jessica G. | | |
| 27. O/S Supervisor<br>a. Saturday (1 day shift)<br>b. Week day (1 evening shift) | | |
| 28. Bed Beeper—NM of day with beeper | | |
| 29. St. Lukes—Nancy D. | | |
| 30. Clinical Coordinator Role—Lula S.<br>Catherine S. | | |
| 31. Pharmacy—Mary | | |
| 32. Laboratory—Ellen | | |
| 33. Radiology—Joe | | |
| 34. Admitting—Karen | | |
| 35. Human Resources—Helen | | |
| 36. Materials Management—Nita | | |
| 37. Clinic: Medicaid process/regulation, general overview—Patty W. | | |

Evaluator's Name _____ Signature _____
             (Print)

Evaluator's Name _____ Signature _____
             (Print)

Evaluator's Name _____ Signature _____
             (Print)

Evaluator's Name _____ Signature _____
             (Print)

_____
Administrative Director Copy

**Continuing Education**

|  | Date |
|---|---|
| 1. | |
| 2. | |
| 3. | |
| 4. | |
| 5. | |
| 6. | |
| 7. | |
| 8. | |
| 9. | |
| 10. | |
| 11. | |
| 12. | |
| 13. | |
| 14. | |
| 15. | |

Administrative Director Signature: _____

Sample Management Tools

# Appendix F

# Satisfaction Surveys

**PATIENT SURVEY**

## PATIENT FOLLOW-UP CALL ♥ ♥ MEDICAL/ SURGICAL FLOORS

*Note to Staff: Please complete all questions (front and back). Any "no" questions must have comments written.*

1. Were you happy with your treatment and care while on either medical or surgical floor?
   Yes ___ No ___
   Comments: _____
   _____
   _____
   _____

2. Was your call light answered in a timely manner?
   Yes ___ No ___

3. Were your requests met in a timely manner? (Such things as pain medication)
   Yes ___ No ___

4. Were you offered assistance before you had to ask? (Such things as getting up to the bathroom or getting fresh water)
   Yes ___ No ___

5. Were the staff members courteous, caring, and compassionate towards you and your family?
   Yes ___ No ___
   Which particular staff members stood out as "exceptional"? Which particular staff member did not appear to meet the standard of friendly, caring, and compassionate?

6. Were you assisted with bathing each morning in a timely manner?
   Yes ___ No ___

## PATIENT FOLLOW-UP CALL ♥♥ MEDICAL/ SURGICAL FLOORS

7. Did the nurses inform you and your family of your plan of care, treatments, and medications before you asked?
   Yes ___ No ___

8. Were your nursing instructions communicated to you clearly?
   Yes ___ No ___

9. At time of discharge, did you feel as though you were given adequate information to go home?
   Yes ___ No ___

10. Did you receive a business card from your nurse informing you of the medical or surgical floor phone number to call if you should have questions or concerns about your condition?
    Yes ___ No ___

11. Are there any other concerns that you would like to share in an effort to help us improve our services?

    _____

    _____

12. Date and Time Called: _____

13. Signature and Title of Caller: _____

Page 2

Sample Management Tools

**PHYSICIAN SURVEY**

## MED/SURG PHYSICIAN SATISFACTION SURVEY

(Individual survey results are strictly confidential)

| Please indicate your level of agreement with the following statements. | Strongly Agree | Agree Somewhat | Disagree Somewhat | Strongly Disagree |
|---|---|---|---|---|
| 1. Overall, DMC is a better place to practice than it was one year ago. Comments: | 4 | 3 | 2 | 1 |
| 2. I believe the quality of patient care on the following area(s) is excellent: A. 3-Central Comments: | 4 | 3 | 2 | 1 |
| B. 3-South Comments: | 4 | 3 | 2 | 1 |
| C. 2-West Comments: | 4 | 3 | 2 | 1 |
| D. Center for Birth Comments: | 4 | 3 | 2 | 1 |
| E. Clinic Comments: | 4 | 3 | 2 | 1 |
| 3. My patients highly rate the quality of care delivered at DMC. Comments: | 4 | 3 | 2 | 1 |

Page 1

## MED/SURG PHYSICIAN SATISFACTION SURVEY

**Please indicate your level of agreement with the following statements.**

| | Strongly Agree | Agree Somewhat | Disagree Somewhat | Strongly Disagree |
|---|---|---|---|---|
| 4. I believe that healthcare providers are customer - friendly in approach to providing services to me as a physician, as well as to my patients. Comments: | 4 | 3 | 2 | 1 |
| 5. Do you have suggestions for the nursing staff for building effective partnerships with physicians and better meeting your needs? If so, please comment as specifically as possible. | | | | |

Thank you for investing your time to assist us in improving our medical/surgical services.

Page 2

# Appendix G

# Critical Pathway Implementation Checklist

---

## CRITICAL PATHWAY IMPLEMENTATION CHECKLIST

Unit: _____          Expected GO-LIVE Date: _____

| Steps | Responsible Persons | Date Due | Date Completed |
|---|---|---|---|
| 1. Choose DRG | | | |
| 2. Research cost and LOS (per physician); generate report to share | | | |
| 3. Obtain HCFA/payor Mean LOS and reimbursement | | | |
| 4. Determine team members (all disciplines should participate in pathway development). | | | |
| 5. Develop the pathway | | | |
| • Chart review for practice pattern (10-12 charts) | | | |
| • Literature review for existing pathways | | | |
| 6. Complete | | | |
| • Preprinted physician orders | | | |
| • Patient's plan of care | | | |
| • Patient education and handouts | | | |
| • Review by staff | | | |
| 7. Develop financial pathway from final draft, if appropriate | | | |
| 8. Meet with key physicians for review/approval and to educate | | | |

---

Courtesy of Mount Carmel Medical Center, Columbus, OH.

Page 1

**CRITICAL PATHWAY IMPLEMENTATION CHECKLIST**

Unit: _____          Expected GO-LIVE Date: _____

| Steps | Responsible Persons | Date Due | Date Completed |
|-------|------------|----------|-----------|
| 9. Staff preparation/buy in<br>• Identify go-live date<br>• Plan inservices on documentation, and specific PI plan | | | |
| 10. Go-Live<br>• Test critical pathway for 24-hours before go-live<br>• Case Managers, educators, and implementation team available as resources on go-live date<br>• Weekly meetings with case managers<br>• Follow-up focus group meetings every 2 weeks and then every month to make revisions. | | | |
| 11. Begin data collection for Performance Improvement plan; Determine monthly variance reporting mechanism | | | |

Modified from: Mount Carmel Medical Center-Columbus, OH.

Page 2

# Appendix H

# Patient Concern Report/ Tracking Record

## PATIENT CONCERN REPORT/TRACKING RECORD

### Patient Problem Report

Date _____

Patient's name _____

Patient's record number _____ Room number _____

Patient's telephone number _____

Patient's home address and home telephone number

_____
(Address)

_____
(City, state, zip code)

_____
(Telephone)

Describe patient's problem or concern. Be specific. Note when, how, and from whom you learned of the problem.

_____

_____

_____

_____

List other persons, services, or departments involved. _____

_____

_____

Describe action taken to solve problem. _____

_____

_____

# Appendix I

# Essential References to Acquire for Personal Library

## (Middle and Executive Management Positions)

Batten, J. (1989). *Tough-minded leadership*. New York: American Management Association.

Block, P. (1996). *Stewardship: Choosing service over self-interest*. San Francisco: Berrett-Koehler Publishers.

Bolman, L. & Deal, T. (1991). *Reframing organizations: Artistry, choice and leadership*. San Francisco: Jossey-Bass Publishers.

Coile, R. (1997). *The five stages of managed care: Strategies for providers, HMOs, and suppliers*. Chicago, IL: Health Administration Press.

Cohen, E. (1996). *Nurse case management in the 21st century*. St. Louis: Mosby.

Covey, S. (1989). *The seven habits of highly effective people: Powerful lessons in personal change*. New York: Simon & Schuster Publishers.

Covey, S. (1991). *Principle-centered leadership*. New York: Simon & Schuster Publishers.

Drucker, P. (1995). *Managing in a time of great change*. New York: Truman Tally Books/Dutton.

Finkler, S. (1992). *Budgeting concepts for nurse managers*. Philadelphia: W.B. Saunders Company.

Ginzberg, E. (1991). *Health services research: Key to health policy*. Cambridge, MA: Harvard University Press.

Katz, J. & Green, E. (1997). *Managing quality*. St. Louis: Mosby.

Kirk, R. (1988). *Healthcare quality and productivity: Practical management tools*. Rockville, MD: Aspen Publishers.

Kirk, R. (1988) *Healthcare staffing and budgeting: Practical management tools*. Rockville, MD: Aspen Publishers.

Pritchett, P. (1997). *Teamwork: The team member handbook*. Dallas, TX: Pritchett & Associates.

Pritchett, P. & Pound, R. (1994). *The employee handbook for organizational change*. Dallas, TX: Pritchett & Associates.

Rowland, H. & Rowland, B. (1995). *Volume 1: Nursing administration manual*. Rockville, MD: Aspen Publishers.

Rowland, H. & Rowland, B. (1995). *Volume 2: Nursing administration manual.* Rockville, MD: Aspen Publishers.

Schroeder, P. (1994). *Improving quality and performance.* St. Louis: Mosby.

Secretan, L. (1997). *Reclaiming higher ground: Creating organizations that inspire the soul.* Toronto: MacMillan Canada Publishing Company.

Senge, P. et. al. (1994). *The fifth discipline fieldbook: Strategies and tools for building a learning organization.* New York: Bantam Doubleday Dell Publishing Group.

Strasen, L. (1987). *Key business skills for nurse managers.* Philadelphia: J.B. Lippincott.

Wolper, L. (1995). *Health care administration: Principles, practices, structure, and delivery.* Gaithersburg, MD: Aspen Publishers.

# Index